Complications

A Doctor's Love Story

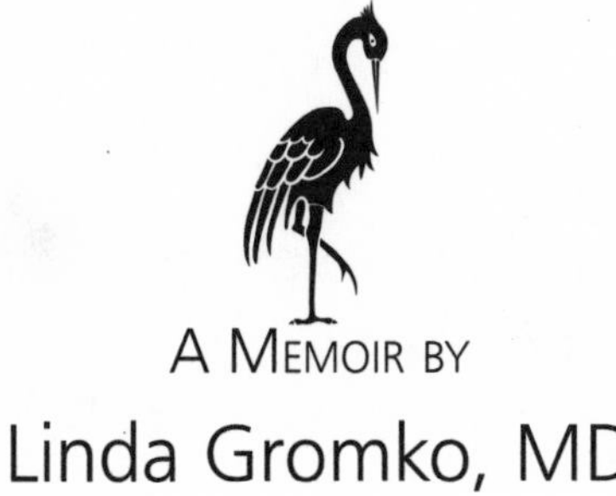

A Memoir by

Linda Gromko, MD

ISBN 978-0-9825143-0-6

Library of Congress Control Number: 2009931866

Linda Gromko MD may be contacted as follows:

www.LindaGromkoMD.com

Mailing Address:
Linda Gromko, MD
200 W. Mercer #104
Seattle, Washington 98119

Note: the above contact information applies to matters of Dr. Gromko's *writing projects only*. Please do not contact her at these addresses for medical advice or for matters pertaining to your own medical care. Thank you.

Disclaimer

Complications: A Doctor's Love Story deals extensively with a variety of medical topics including diabetes, kidney disease, heart disease, and abnormalities of the blood.

While the book is intended to inform and entertain, it is not intended to be a substitute for seeking your own medical advice from your personal health care provider.

If my book raises questions about your own health, seek one-on-one care for your answers. There's a saying: "The patient who treats himself/herself has a fool for a doctor."

Now that the Internet has offered a deluge of medical information, I always tell my own patients, "Double-click on judgment!" Seek professional advice about matters as important as your life and health.

Linda Gromko, MD

Dedication

This book is dedicated to my loving husband,
Stephen Martin Williams,
And to our children,
Tim Franklin
And
Brita Williams

Who, in full collaboration, have taught me more about love
Than I would have ever thought possible!

About the Cover

The beautiful cover of *Complications: A Doctor's Love Story* was designed by Seattle's Bob Bost. Bob started by photographing the Asian screen, one of the actual items included in Jeff Milner's bequest to Linda Gromko. His photograph of the breathtaking screen was then wrapped around the book to feature the image of the Asian cranes—traditional symbols of wisdom and longevity.

Bob Bost works as a graphic designer in Seattle. His personal interests are broad, and he is passionate about promoting healing through music. Bob participates in a Seattle musicians' group which brings live music to patients in area hospitals. A prolific songwriter, he has written haunting and inspirational works such as *On Christmas Morn, Friend's Waltz, and Fight the Good Fight.*

Preface

As a family doctor in Seattle, I have owned and operated a small medical clinic since 1989. I have learned that running an independent family practice requires a continual flirtation with chaos; the only real constant is that I never know what might happen from one moment to the next.

My staff of ten, including three first-rate nurse practitioners, serves a full spectrum of folks from the destitute to the privileged. Our clients deal with the range of life's challenges: untamed children, aging parents, alcoholism, gender asynchrony, financial stresses, relationship and career dilemmas, and a full mélange of medical problems. If anything, however, we attract well meaning people who seek to contribute to the world in some way or another—people who seem compelled to make a difference.

My own life has long been driven by a compulsion to right the wrongs I've perceived. Even as a high school student in the sixties, I lobbied in our state capital for the eighteen-year-old vote. I served as the editor of my high school newspaper—as well as the editor of our alternative free press rag, *The Antidote.* As a student nurse, I discovered that working at the local free clinic brought far more personal meaning than my formal studies at the University of Washington School of

Nursing. While a nurse practitioner at Planned Parenthood, I championed reproductive freedoms and learned first-hand about the responsibility of patient advocacy.

In my early days as a staff physician, I worked to ban smoking in my hospital—a cause that seems unthinkable now, but most assuredly ruffled the feathers of the old guard. I poured tireless hours into vocal advocacy for Washington State's Physician Aid-In-Dying campaign in 1990, publicly debating physicians who were far more credentialed than I was. Tilting at windmills had always been a bit of a specialty for me. And calling out a naked emperor now and then seemed as natural to me as breathing.

While fighting the professional battles comes naturally, fighting my *own* battles has always been trickier. Like many of my physician colleagues, I have struggled to perfect a sense of balance: finding meaning in my professional life while still nurturing meaningful personal relationships; aching to incorporate recreational activities into the ever-expanding work. For me, balance has been hard to achieve.

Yet now and again, circumstances *insist* that we find our footing—or fall away. Such was my predicament in the spring of 2004, when I received an implausible inheritance from a former patient.

The experiences that followed provided the imperative to reexamine my life's priorities and affirm my own needs. Finding my true life partner and then witnessing his precipitous fall into the hell of acute kidney failure allowed me to assert my most powerful advocacy yet: I learned to fight for the love of my life, and for my own life as well.

Chapter One

One Tuesday in the spring of 2004, I rushed out of my medical office to meet my friend Connie for lunch. It was time for our mutual therapy session: lunch at Seattle's Pacific Place.

Connie and I had been friends since our pre-med classes twenty-five years before. In medical school, the two of us were members of a support group for nurses who were training to become physicians. When we graduated, we continued to get together almost monthly for lunch or dinner—as a support group of only two. Over the decades, we tracked each other through births and deaths, and my two divorces.

Noble and creative work, the practice of medicine filled my life, but it also insulated me from seeking a new primary relationship after my second marriage failed in 1996. There was always a work project or a woman in labor to shield me from getting hurt again. Yet, I always yearned for a man who would become my friend and mate for life.

I learned that an independent medical practice is a complicated small business. Like housework or parenting, the work can expand to occupy all conceivable time available. Sometimes it seemed like I did nothing but work and sleep, although after many years, I cultivated a healthy addiction to physical exercise. My meetings with Connie were likewise a necessity; we both needed to laugh and let go of the stresses of our busy lives.

On that particular spring day in 2004 as I was preparing to meet Connie for lunch, I received a call from the King County Coroner's Office. Physicians receive such calls from time to time, usually to provide details about a patient who had died unexpectedly.

"Dr. Gromko, this is Nick Foster. I'm an investigator with the King County Coroner's Office. I'm calling about Jeffrey Milner (not his real name)—a sixty-year-old male who passed at his apartment three days ago."

"Milner," I said. "You know, I'm not sure who you're talking about. Could you give me some more information about this man?"

With minimal prompting, I resurrected the memory of my former patient: a too-slender, but immaculately appointed gentleman, usually wearing white linen trousers and carrying a leather attaché case. Jeff was eccentric, fussy and demanding, but always polite.

Jeff's problems were enormous—medical, financial, social, and psychiatric. He would arrive at our medical office long before his scheduled appointments, and expect our staff to devote hours to him. Jeff could have utilized a full staff—just for him. As with all of our patients, my staff and I sincerely tried to help. I remembered giving Jeff my own family recipes for healthy diabetic-friendly meals which could work on a limited fixed income. We truly spent hours with Jeff, but our efforts were never enough.

Ultimately, we felt obliged to ask him to find a larger practice, recommending that he seek care from the University of Washington Medical Center—a place where he could have his specialists and the benefit of psychiatric and social services all under one roof. In the trade, we call this "finding a better therapeutic match." Sometimes this serves as sort of a "dishonorable discharge" when issues of rudeness or abuse surface, or when a patient refuses to pay a legitimate bill. Such issues did not apply to Jeff, however. He was simply too much for our little practice to accommodate. We almost never discharged patients from my practice!

"I *do* remember Jeff," I explained to the investigator, "but he hasn't been to my office in years. How did he die?"

"Oh, he died of natural causes," the investigator explained, "and another doctor has already signed the death certificate. That's not why

I'm calling."

I was getting curious.

"I'm calling because Mr. Milner designated you as his beneficiary."

I now cringed at the thought of having discharged Jeff from the practice.

"But I haven't seen him in probably ten years," I said. "Isn't there a family member or someone else who would be more appropriate?"

"We've looked, and there's no family," replied the investigator. "But this happens all the time. People die, with no friends or family. And they leave everything to somebody who's done them a kindness somewhere along the line.

"Now you should understand that Mr. Milner lived in public housing, and he wasn't a wealthy man—but he had a lot of really nice stuff. And if you don't claim it, it'll all be thrown away. I think you should go and take a look."

I agreed to claim Mr. Milner's personal effects, meeting the investigator at the county morgue at Harborview Medical Center. There was a wallet with a photo ID that matched my memory; there might have been a dozen credit cards, a few personal papers, and a key to the Capitol Park Apartment unit Jeff had occupied.

I accepted the personal items stuffed into a brown paper shopping bag, and paid the $140 fee which would cover Mr. Milner's internment—a no-frills cremation with burial in the local "Potter's Field." It would be a pauper's burial, but a burial nonetheless. And it seemed the appropriate thing to do, after all.

The investigator asked me again when I'd last seen Jeff; our medical charting verified that we hadn't seen him in *fifteen years!*

"Well, that *is* interesting," said Mr. Foster, pointing to the form from the Seattle Housing Authority.

"See here," he said, "'On my death, all my personal belongings go to Dr. Linda Gromko.' It was signed in September of 2003—*seven months before he died.* It was a recent bequest."

Chapter Two

I enlisted the help of my office manager and friend Barb Boni in this curious project. We sifted through Jeff's papers: a birth certificate, a passport, and a letter of reference from Jeff's last landlord before he moved to Capitol Park. There were letters pertaining to his travels abroad, vouching for a teaching position he'd held in Austria.

Then, we found four envelopes with multiple three-by-five-inch photographs: photo-documentation of Jeff's possessions. It was the type of photo inventory you might provide for your homeowner's insurance company in case of theft or damage.

Barb and I scanned through the pictures. One envelope contained detailed photos of serving platters, dishes, and kitchen equipment—two standing Kitchen Aid mixers and restaurant-sized stock pots. Jeff had over a dozen LeCruset pieces—the type of cookware you'd buy at Williams and Sonoma—in an array of vibrant colors.

Another envelope contained pictures of Jeff's closet: a dozen high-end bathrobes, numerous pairs of shoes, and multiple leather jackets perfectly arranged as if displayed at Nordstrom. The "Office Envelope" featured Jeff's computer equipment, and an assortment of ornate fountain pens precisely laid out in a parallel fashion, possibly collectors' items. A fourth envelope detailed Jeff's living room—bookcases stuffed floor-to-ceiling with coffee table art books, vases, clocks, decorative plates, and statues of the Buddha.

"Well, this is pretty unbelievable," I said to Barb. "Please—you have to go with me and see what this is all about."

Barb agreed, and we contacted the Seattle Housing Authority building manager. He assured me that the bequest was valid, and that there was no family. Furthermore, the manager confirmed that if I didn't come and take Mr. Milner's items, they would all be discarded. The manager advised us to telephone a man named David (not his real name), Mr. Milner's designated contact person. David would give us a key card to let us into the building.

It was a rainy April afternoon when Barb and I made our way up to Capitol Park. As we buzzed David's unit, a Medic One crew meandered by us, transporting a tattooed man on a gurney. He'd reportedly had a seizure, but he was fully lucid and talking without difficulty, specifying his preferred doctor at Harborview. Another man with a raggedy gray beard scurried by us in a tie-dyed tank top and a purple chiffon skirt.

Then, a middle-aged woman approached us. She was wearing a navy blue sweatshirt, shorts, and turquoise anklets without shoes.

"I'm Sister Mary Catherine," she said, extending her hand to Barb and then to me. "How can I help you?"

We explained that we were looking for David, Jeff Milner's friend, and Sister Mary Catherine volunteered eagerly to take us to David's apartment.

"So you are Jeff's family," said Sister Mary Catherine, leading us down a corridor with linoleum floors so polished they looked like marble—at least from a distance.

"No, Sister," I replied. "Jeff was actually a patient of mine, a very long time ago. What Order are you associated with?"

"The Sisters of the Holy Cross," she said, "but I have been living here since the aneurysm . . . in my brain."

Sister Mary Catherine knocked on David's door, then introduced Barb and me to a middle-aged man with a touch of strabismus resulting in a mildly wandering left eye. He invited us to enter his apartment unit, immaculately tidy but heavy with the smell of cigarette smoke.

We spoke of Jeff's death. No one had seen him for several days;

David said Jeff had been having trouble with his diabetes, and had lost a lot of weight recently. A woman in the apartment next door to Jeff had heard some thumping noises on Good Friday; she told David that something had been going on in the "spirit world." The coroner had thought Jeff probably *had* died on Good Friday, though his body was removed from the apartment a few days later.

David, Barb, and I chatted for a few moments. I explained to David how perplexed I was that Jeff had designated me as his beneficiary. He maintained that Jeff had spoken of me as his physician quite recently.

I shook my head, and David sighed.

"Dr. Gromko, there is something I think you should know about Jeff."He paused.

"Well, first of all, Jeff was gay."

"Well, that doesn't matter to me, David," I said.

"And then, there's this. . . ." he paused again, "Jeff really liked watching porn videos. And he had a huge collection."

"Well, okay," I said. None of this seemed as weighty as David was making it.

"Would you like to have it?"

David lit up.

"Yes!" he exclaimed.

We had made our first dispersal of Jeff's "remainders."

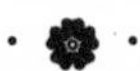

The Capitol Park Apartment was home to a motley collection of individuals who had tumbled off life's grid in one way or another. We would learn that most were terribly poor, and many had disabilities—physical and/or mental—which made them ineligible to participate in the mainstream of life. The rent was cheap, $166 per month for Jeff's eleventh-floor penthouse unit.

But it became achingly apparent to us that the admission price was very steep indeed. You had to "qualify" to live there by having literally no other options. It was a marginal step above homelessness.

The idea that Jeff's things would have been simply discarded—if

I did nothing—was untenable. Surely, someone could use his things; there were many charities to benefit. David suggested an AIDS charity, and I thought immediately of Lambert House—a drop-in center for gay, lesbian, bisexual, and transgendered youth. I knew the center needed money. Furthermore, my practice served a substantial number of transgendered patients.

Still puzzled as to why I had received this windfall, I figured I could at least serve as a responsible steward of Jeff's possessions. Through my advocacy, Jeff's things might benefit the larger community.

Barb and I entered Jeff's apartment later that afternoon. We could barely force the door open; the tiny place was so crammed full of books, furniture, and a mammoth audiovisual entertainment center.

"Oh my God!" I gasped, nearly overcome by the smell. The stench was unimaginable: a combination of spoiled food, Patchouli oil, dust, feces, and urine—and the lingering scent of a dead body, now removed, which had occupied the unit for several days.

"Look at all this stuff, Linda," coughed Barb, sputtering in response to the particulate matter floating about.

We could see at a glance that the small apartment was divided into an entry hall, a closet-sized kitchen, a living room, and a small bedroom with adjoining bath.

The sheer quantity of "things" was staggering—far more than would be required by any single individual. There was enough "stuff" for many families. We discovered specific categories of things. Jeff had a lamp "department," for example, and ultimately, a total of thirteen separate Oriental rugs stacked one on top of another. The art books were beautiful; floor-to-ceiling shelves of coffee table volumes from the Metropolitan Museum of Art. Many were still packaged in their original cellophane wrappers, never opened and never read. Jeff's CD collection numbered in the hundreds, featuring packaged sets of classical music and opera. Once again, many were unopened.

We simply had to stop and absorb what Jeff had left. The project of sorting, discarding, and donating the goods was going to take time. We left, knowing we needed reinforcements to help us.

I phoned my friend, Steve Mitchell, to describe my odd inheritance. Dr. Mitchell was a practicing psychiatrist with both an MD and a PhD degree. I would kid him that his excessive education made him far too smart for the rest of us mortals. He was clearly a genius, though he would never reveal his IQ. Like most highly intelligent people, Dr. Mitchell had an insatiable curiosity—and Jeff's apartment was a forensic mother lode. He agreed to meet Barb and me to survey Jeff's possessions.

This time, Barb and I came prepared with surgical masks, latex examination gloves, and black plastic lawn bags for trash. After a brief orientation for Dr. Mitchell, the three of us set about the task of sorting items and discarding obvious garbage.

Barb started working in the kitchen, scrubbing spoiled food off the counters and emptying the refrigerator. There wasn't much food in the refrigerator; food stamps don't buy a full pantry. Jeff, however, did stock a cabinet with odds and ends he'd obviously bought in bulk: Cups-o-Noodles, cans of soup, boxes of seasoned rice mixes. We decided to take these items to a table in the first floor Common Room. Capitol Park residents scooped them up instantly, scurrying back to their units to secure their treasures. Jeff's cleaning products also vanished from the Common Room table, and unopened rolls of toilet paper might as well have been gold. Food stamps do not cover cleaning items or sundries.

Dr. Mitchell and I started to tackle the bedroom and adjoining bathroom. The odor was stifling, but Steve suggested we begin by removing the bed linens. Jeff's body had been removed only a week before, and the bed was still damp from bodily fluids. I gagged as we tugged the sheets off the bed and stuffed them into a plastic trash bag. I, who delivered fifty babies every year, was nearly over the bucket with nausea. My colleague—the psychiatrist—took it all in stride.

Bit by bit, we began to sort. We discovered that Jeff was a catalogue shopper, and that he had excellent taste. But what he demonstrated in style, he lacked in decisiveness. Jeff would order not *one* polo shirt, but six polo shirts—presumably one in each color available. There were multiples of angora sweaters and scarves—again, each item represented in various colors. Jeff loved leather goods: gloves, briefcases, belts, and wallets. He fancied monogrammed items. His bathrobes and smoking jackets were flamboyant and expensive. There were a dozen classic woolen and leather jackets. It was apparent that Jeff purchased items in keeping with the manner in which he defined himself: elegant, educated, and refined.

We found towels: not the threadbare kind I had in my home, but lush, thirsty Egyptian cotton towels—again in a rainbow of colors. As with his books, and music collection, many of the towels were brand new.

Dr. Mitchell stopped me at one point.

"So what are you going to take home today?" he asked.

"Well, this isn't mine, Steve. I mean, I'm going to give it away."

"It *is* yours. It is *all* yours. Why don't you start by choosing something to take with you today?"

Dr. Mitchell's point—that the windfall was mine—made me uncomfortable. Perhaps the bequest had been a mistake on Jeff's part; after all, I *had* discharged him from my practice. Certainly, there was no honor in "expelling" Jeff. Perhaps it was an odd joke; I really didn't know what to make of it. But there was no doubt that I felt more at ease in giving everything away than in receiving *anything* at all. I was a woman who tended to downplay birthdays and Christmas for myself, and Valentine flowers would come from my son, not from a lover.

I looked around and found a carved wooden fish, a hummingbird mobile, and several unopened boxes of note cards from the Metropolitan Museum of Art. I liked the whimsical look of the fish and the mobile, and I tended to write a lot of thank-you notes.

"Okay," I said hastily, "I'll take these. But you and Barb have to take some things, too. We are *all* working on this project!"

Barb chose a couple of beautiful LeCruset casseroles, and Dr. Mitchell claimed the collection of fountain pens. We ended our day by deciding that we would continue working on the project, each selecting things we knew we would genuinely enjoy. There would be so much left; we would barely make a dent by taking our few selections.

During our next day at Capitol Park, Barb, Dr. Mitchell, and I became more acquainted with Jeff's art collection. The classic Leonardo daVinci figure drawing which hung over Jeff's bed was later to find a home over my condominium fireplace. There were many prints—nothing terribly expensive, but all sophisticated and tasteful. A series of three Asian princes hung vertically at the far end of the apartment. Jeff had several wooden clocks: detailed creations with musical chimes to mark the hours we spent in his abode.

We sorted through hundreds of fine books, dividing them into categories: art, literature, music, cookbooks, and travel. Among the volumes, Jeff had arranged several sets of candlesticks, Metropolitan Museum of Art bookends, and fifteen Buddha statues.

Our furniture inventory included a substantial wooden bed, two dining tables with coordinating dining chairs, a green leather chair and ottoman from Dania, six lamps, several ornamental mirrors, five giant bookcases, a teak bedroom cabinet, two work desks, and a complete outfit of computer equipment. The massive entertainment center had already been removed—given to David to enhance the value of Jeff's coveted pornography collection.

We also found paper grocery bags of old, unused prescription medications: antidepressants, anxiety pills, and narcotics, which never found their intended recipient. But the specific drugs allowed us to speculate on Jeff's diagnoses: depression, obsessive-compulsive disorder, generalized anxiety disorder perhaps. The three of us flushed the medicines down the toilet, though we commented that the salable street drugs and the pornography collection would have netted a hefty sum.

Finally, tucked in between the apartment wall and a floor-to-ceiling bookcase, we found what was for me the most striking discovery of all. I had been looking for a decorative Asian screen for years. Discreetly hidden and still wrapped in its original packing material was one of the most stunning Asian screens I had ever seen! Its four adjoining panels featured six white cranes poised on a golden background. A subtle underlying pattern of repeating squares replicated the tiles surrounding my home fireplace. The heads of the cranes precisely matched the saddle leather of my couch, and the sage fir and bamboo trees in the background complemented my upholstered easy chair. No decorator could have hand-picked a more perfect accessory for my family room.

It was as though Jeff had selected the Asian screen for me, and me alone. I was beginning to entertain the notion that this inheritance *was* purposefully bestowed. I stepped up to become the keeper of the cranes, these ancient symbols of wisdom and longevity. Rescued from Jeff's obscurity, the cranes went to my home that afternoon—fitting perfectly in a place of honor.

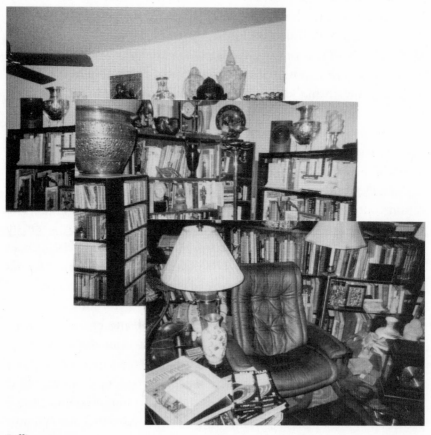

Jeff's apartment

Later, I phoned the head of Lambert House to see if they might welcome contributions from our curious benefactor. The drop-in center for sexual-minority youth was preparing for its annual garage sale, and would send volunteers with a truck to help us distribute our wealth.

The volunteer crew was headed by a good-natured gentleman in his twenties, displaying more tattoo art per square centimeter of body surface area than I had ever seen. He brought his own reinforcements, in the form of two other gentlemen, and a large U-haul truck preparing for a day's work.

Truckload after truckload ventured out from the Capitol Park Apartments, heading to Lambert House for further sorting. Ultimately, Jeff's things occupied half of the area of the St. Joseph's School auditorium where the annual Lambert House fundraiser was held. It was truly amazing; Dr. Mitchell and I watched as people gathered up their treasures—with just a hint of the scent of Jeff's apartment lingering in the air.

Back at Capitol Park, Barb and I gave the apartment a final cleaning. Now empty, the unit seemed quite spacious. We wiped down the picture windows: windows we could barely see with all the clutter of Jeff's life. The view spanned all of downtown Seattle, the glorious Seattle waterfront, and the majestic snow-capped peak of Mount Rainier.

I stopped, my body shuddering momentarily. To the core of my being, I recognized that Jeff had sent an ethereal message. Jeff's unwritten, unspoken message was directed, personal, and clear. And the message *was* for me:

If your life is encumbered to the point where you miss the best parts available—even if the encumbrances are positive, it is time to re-examine your priorities, redirect your energies, and discover the gifts that are intended for you!

Here we were in an apartment so encumbered that we couldn't appreciate the most beautiful feature it offered: the view. In my *life,* I was so busy trying to meet everyone else's needs: never missing a labor pain—let alone a delivery! While I loved my work, the most precious thing of all—a significant relationship with a wonderful man to love as an equal partner—had always eluded me.

It was time to rearrange my life: time for rowing, time to write, time to find a partner, time to live *my life.* Of course I didn't elect to leave medicine. Medicine is a crucial piece of who I am. But I did decide to stop delivering babies—without question, one of the favorite chapters of my medical career. And I decided to learn to practice medicine in a more balanced way that would allow me to continue serving people without building the resentment that grows from self-neglect.

The "Jeff Experience" brought many other lessons, too. Use the new towels! Listen to the CDs! Read the books! Appreciate the abundance we all have—simply by being alive! We don't always need more *things* to live richly.

The "Jeff Experience" presented several tests for me. Would I receive his message? I did. Would I act on the message? I have. Would I demonstrate to the universe my ability to serve as a responsible steward of life's gifts? Yes, and I was later to be awarded far more valuable gifts than I ever would have expected—all because of Jeff.

Chapter Three

Still reeling from the apparent blessing from the Universe, I set out in earnest to find a life partner. While I had tried before, I never seemed to "get it right." And it was truly the only regret in my life. Why could other people find happiness with a partner, but not me? It was time to try again, and I intended to proceed efficiently!

"Big and Beefy," my personal trainer at the time, took a couple of photos of me: a head shot at a party, and an informal pose with me perched on a spinning bike wearing my exercise clothing and a baseball cap. They weren't glamour shots to be sure, but they showed a real person.

I opened an account on Match.com, posted the photos, and announced to the world: "I'd like to meet a nice Democrat." The rest of my profile explained that I had a grown son, worked in healthcare, didn't smoke or drink, had allergies to cats and dogs, didn't want kids, loved movies, and spent my limited spare time in the gym or rowing.

My ad brought responses from a few non-felons, and I began to date. Then, I received a "wink"—the Match.com notation conveying interest—from a man nicknamed "Bugdad" with the header "on an island, just a boat ride to the city."

Steve Williams, who lived a ferry ride away on nearby Bainbridge Island with his nine-year-old daughter Brita ("the Bug"), described himself as follows:

> *A devoted father with an abundant capacity for more fun in our scene as well as an interest in a great woman for fun as a couple. Character with humor and warmth is what I have and expect.*
>
> *I would enjoy a woman who is alive of intellect, liberal of politics, reads to explore and imagine, knows what three sets of ten means, and has a wide spectrum of acceptance for the behavior of friends.*

Three sets of ten! This was a weight-lifting reference. One woman wrote to Steve, "three sets of ten are thirty." She didn't make the cut!

When Steve "winked" at me in the fall of 2004, I was dating another man—a highly intellectual mathematician who lived in a tiny studio apartment just down the street from the gym of my personal trainer. We shared a number of common interests: mostly physical training and movies. But it grew clear to me that one of our most pressing common interests was him! One evening, this gentleman hosted a dinner gathering for four of his closest friends. The intellectual pissing contest between the men, and a slide show complete with a photo of his drop-dead-gorgeous and *maybe-former* girlfriend grew too much for me to tolerate.

I said "Good night and good-bye," and got back on Match.com the next day.

For some reason, I remembered "Bugdad." This was curious because I hadn't written down his moniker, and even more curious because of the fact that Bugdad *was* a dad. My "baby son" was twenty-eight at the time, and I certainly wasn't looking for any new children. I winked at "Bugdad" anyway.

> *You may recall you winked at me some time ago; I was dating a man at the time and wanted to see how it would play out. (It played out.) I was attracted to your profile because of the reference to how you want your daughter treated, and to*

your Queen Anne High School alum status, as I am a Queen Anne High alum as well.

I am a feminist prochoice family practice physician in solo practice with three nurse practitioners. I deliver a lot of babies, though I will be ending the baby business in April. I expect that it will be a big adjustment, so therapists are standing by! I do a range of medical services, including treatment of Seattle's transgendered community.

Personally, I have a twenty-eight-year-old son who lives in Montana, working as a sportscaster. I spend much of my free time doing spin cycling and rowing with the Lake Washington Rowing Club. If the above disclaimers don't worry you, please write back. I would like to hear more about your work and your daughter.

After about a week of e-mailing, Steve and I met for the first time at a Queen Anne Starbucks. I recognized him from his photo on Match.com: fair of complexion with thinning blond hair. Actually, there was very little hair on the top of his head at all except for a patch of corn-silk, which Steve combed straight back; I was relieved that it was not a comb-over. He had engaging blue eyes and a pair of reading glasses perched atop his forehead. Steve was notably broad through the shoulders, balancing a full belly—lending credence to his stated background in fitness. It was easy to see that he might have been a power lifter some years in the past.

Steve was tastefully dressed in a finely knit Merino wool black sweater, bone wide-wale cords, Italian leather shoes, and a silver Rolex. I would learn during our coffee date that his toney sweater would catch dribbles of coffee, but I would also learn that this man was more invested in our tender new conversation than he was in coffee drippings.

Steve leaned into the conversation. He wanted to know about my life's chronology, starting from my early childhood and moving on through my career. He wanted to know about my family, how I got along with my parents, and whom we might have known in common over the years. He was a gentle interrogator, a thoughtful listener. His eyes were kind; his easy smile and ready banter skillfully drew me in. He learned a great deal about me in less than an hour, but he was eager to share his own information so I never felt overly exposed.

As it turned out, Steve and I had gone to the same high school, graduating only two years apart. One of his best friends was George Mead, whose father, George Mead Sr., had been my math teacher in junior high. Steve and I had attended the same concerts on the same days. The commonalities, the parallels in our non-intersecting lives, were notable. Steve had even been married to the sister of a medical school classmate of mine. We had both left fractured relationships years before.

I learned that Steve was a consultant to two separate industries: home electronics and personal fitness. He had owned several companies including the locally infamous (i.e. "colorful") Speakerlab, and had traveled internationally on business.

He was widely read, irreverently funny, and gifted at banter. Politically and socially liberal, Steve was a man who "did the right thing." He claimed to be "loyal as a beagle" and agreed with my requirement for an "infidelity death pact." Our priorities matched; our chemistry clicked.

The coffee date flowed on into dinner. I probably startled Steve by asking him for results of his STD (Sexually Transmitted Disease) screens on our first date. But, hey, the guy had me at "wink."

Over the next three years, Steve and I forged ahead with a tender new relationship. It wasn't always easy. We could antagonize each other with a look, and our arguments were messy. We were clearly both "bosses" in our own right, not accustomed to compromise in our personal lives. But our deep comfort with each other and our commitment to each other were automatic. We *knew* we were each other's right partner.

Like most relationships, however, ours was complicated. First of all, I had never envisioned finding a partner with a young child. Brita was nine years old when I met her. And Steve had had full custody of her—by court order—from the time she was only two. Steve and Brita were a package deal.

I hadn't sought out the complexities of parenting again, having raised Tim, in part, as a single parent. But even more than the messiness of parenting, I felt the moral imperative of avoiding *anything* that would injure Brita. I remember telling Steve on our first date, "I promise you I won't hurt your daughter."

Partly because he was a single parent, Steve had chosen to raise Brita on Bainbridge Island, a well-to-do island community with a superior public school system. And "only a thirty-five-minute ferry ride to Seattle!" Truly, on a sunlit vacation day, the ferry ride was the stuff of brochures. But on a daily basis, the grinding Bainbridge commute ate up two to three hours a day: rushing, waiting, and riding on what I referred to only as "that fucking boat."

Even before our relationship began, I was juggling many demands: my medical practice with its patients and personnel; the non-negotiable, yet reasonable requirements of my eighty-nine-year-old mother; the details of a couple of rental properties. My son Tim was grown, and on his own—but close enough to help and to need help on occasion too. I clung to my personal therapies of rowing and spin cycling, and maintained relationships with a handful of longtime friends like Connie and Dr. Mitchell—all of which required their own time and logistics.

My medical practice required an enormous investment of time and energy. I had established my family medical practice in Seattle twenty years earlier. Started from scratch, "one Pap at a time," I had nursed it through financially thin and nearly desperate times—more than once charging the payroll for my ten staff members to the VISA card. For many years, the practice loan was secured by my home. But it was a true labor of love: delivering hundreds of babies, shepherding my special transgendered clients through their intricate transitions, and generally serving a diversity of individuals who trusted *me* with the privileged intimacies of their lives, their most precious secrets.

For the first two years of my relationship with Steve, I straddled Seattle and Bainbridge Island. It was a logistical nightmare; every detail of my life requiring precise orchestration. A missed ferry could be disastrous, throwing my usually busy life into further chaos.

Yet, even logic wouldn't allow me to shake the feeling that this relationship was worth the trouble. After all, it had flowed so naturally out of Jeff's implausible gift. Furthermore, I had made a promise to stay in the game and never—*never* to harm Brita.

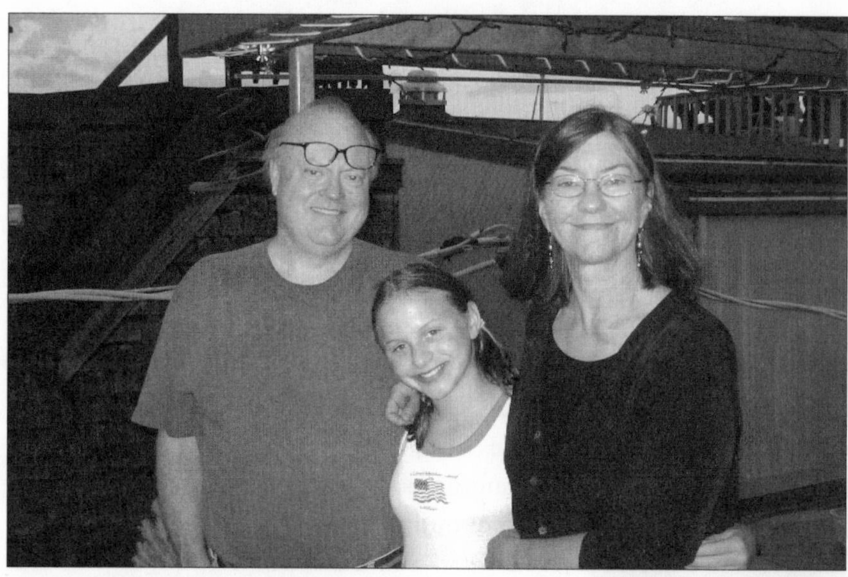

Steve, daughter Brita, and Linda at Carol Frieberg's fourth of July gathering on a houseboat on Seattle's Lake Union, 2006 (Photo by Carol Frieberg)

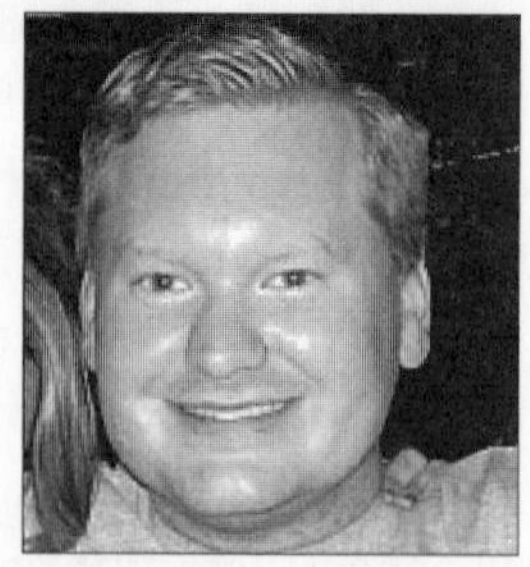

Tim Franklin (Linda's son)

Chapter Four

Another—and far more consequential—issue in our relationship was Steve's health. When I met him, I recognized Steve as a lovable poster child for what is medically known as "metabolic syndrome": a combination of high blood pressure, abnormal cholesterol and triglycerides, elevated blood sugar, and that visible extra weight around the middle. This complex of conditions greatly increases a person's risk for cardiovascular diseases like stroke and heart attack.

People have asked me why I even considered a relationship with a man with these potential health problems. The fact is, however, we *all* have—or will have—health problems. Particularly as a physician, I recognized the capricious nature of who gets into medical trouble and who doesn't. It's never that clear. What *was* clear to me, however, was that Steve Williams wasn't the kind of man you passed up. He was my partner, and I knew early in the game that I was in it for the duration—whatever that might mean.

When I first met Steve, his hemoglobin AlC, a reflection of blood sugar over the prior three months, was a frightfully high ten percent (normal is less than six). Steve had adult onset diabetes mellitus; he'd known it for years and reluctantly took oral medications to try to manage it. With some nudging on my part, Steve acquiesced to starting on insulin. This brought his blood sugars down into a more reasonable, safer range.

But the diabetes had already begun to take its toll. The "death of a thousand cuts," as Steve's doctor put it; diabetes affects both large blood vessels and tiny blood vessels in the body. Large vessels, for example, are those of the heart. Steve had already had a coronary artery bypass graft (CABG—or "cabbage" in the trade) at age fifty. Thankfully, the blockages in his heart vessels were suspected during a screening EKG; he had not actually had a heart attack or heart muscle damage. But the surgery had been complicated by a massive staphylococcal infection requiring a second surgery to re-open his chest and drain out the pus. Steve had to self-administer IV vancomycin by way of a PICC line ("peripherally inserted central catheter") for a period of six months, even on transoceanic flights. Brita had been only four years old at that time.

The diabetes had also affected the tiny blood vessels in Steve's eyes; he had had two retinal surgeries years before we met. Little nerves in the legs and feet were impacted, producing a numbing, discomfiting condition called "peripheral neuropathy." Diabetics often experience foot ulcers and amputations of digits, simply because they cannot feel the day-to-day injuries the rest of us notice. I would remove a rock from a shoe or straighten out a wrinkle in my sock, for example. In a diabetic, however, such minor insults could go unnoticed and develop into non-healing, limb-threatening wounds.

Steve had also experienced a diabetic complication where he had suddenly lost all feeling in his left leg. While it had improved to some degree, the leg was still unreliable. Steve had difficulty with "proprioception," the ability to tell where his left leg was in relation to things around him. This made his gait unreliable, particularly in the dark or when he was tired. He looked wobbly, but rarely fell.

By the time the eyes and peripheral nerves are involved, most diabetics have some degree of kidney disease. I suspect that this is an aspect of diabetes of which the general public knows very little. Yet we were to learn that diabetic kidney disease was one of the most relentless enemies Steve would face, and I would face with him.

Chapter Five

I learned about kidneys in medical school, and before that, in nursing school, although you never absorb concepts as fully as when *your* life and love are so directly impacted.

Kidneys are complicated; they have a variety of functions. Good kidney function is a requirement for good health, and poor kidney function steals it away. We all know that our kidneys make urine. In the process, they filter out toxins from the blood and squeeze out the body's excess fluid. They also make EPO, a hormone that stimulates the bone marrow to produce red blood cells. The kidneys convert inactive Vitamin D into an active form, which facilitates proper calcium absorption and normal bone health. They produce renin, a hormone which helps to regulate blood pressure.

So when kidneys don't work well, you can see a variety of symptoms. In its early stages, kidney disease may have no symptoms at all. Later symptoms may include bloating, mental fogginess, itching, bone problems, weakness, shortness of breath, and fatigue. Abnormal kidneys can cause high blood pressure and, in turn, high blood pressure can damage kidneys. As kidneys fail, people don't feel well and they don't look healthy. The symptoms can be insidious—creeping up slowly until a person is a little less "present," a little less whole.

While Steve experienced the "creep-up" symptoms for years, he suddenly got very sick very fast—a free-fall into a pit that really might have swallowed him up for good. His kidneys had been quietly worsening, principally as a result of the "usual suspects": diabetes and hypertension (high blood pressure). But he suddenly came down with a severe sinus infection. And a tooth that had bothered him for years flared with a painful abscess. A couple of courses of antibiotics later, Steve was still worsening. He bloated with dozens of extra pounds from a weight of 235 to 270. His tongue swelled and he bit it repeatedly, dulling his enunciation. That, along with a mental fogginess, made him sound less "crisp," almost drunk. I worried that his business colleagues might think him inebriated.

I struggled to avoid serving as Steve's physician, but I could see that he was in urgent trouble. Compulsively, I ordered lab tests. In the world of renal failure, we focus on a chemical called "creatinine." Creatinine is a breakdown product of muscle cells. We continually produce creatinine, and healthy kidneys eliminate it in the urine. The kidneys—in health—hold in sugar molecules and protein, and get rid of creatinine. Steve's sick kidneys poured out massive amounts of protein, and his serum creatinine started to climb. From a worrisome baseline of 2.6 milligrams per deciliter (normal being around 1.0), Steve's creatinine crept up to 4.1. Then, it shot up to his maximum of 10.2 over an astonishing two-week period. Another significant test, the "eGFR" (estimated glomerular filtration rate), plummeted to 5.2 milliliters per minute, with a normal eGFR being well over sixty!

During that time, I was afraid to leave Steve alone. He grew more unsteady, and his body started to get twitchy. With his arms outstretched and his wrists flexed upward, Steve's hands would flap repeatedly, exhibiting a medical phenomenon called "asterixis." Asterixis implies a hyper-excitability of the nervous system, and can occur in circumstances of liver dysfunction, low oxygen levels, and renal impairment. It was an ominous sign of encephalopathy: toxins poisoning the brain.

Steve's nephrologist, the usually jovial Dr. Smiley Thakur, explained that he was experiencing acute renal failure. Dr. Thakur admitted Steve directly to the Swedish Hospital Emergency Room. Sitting in the ER playing "Hangman" with me to pass the time, Steve looked bloated, yellow-gray, and scared to death. His speech was thick; the content was loopy but funny. Ironically, he lost our Hangman game on the word "urination." The ER doctors noted his lab numbers to be "impressive" (a euphemism for "awful"). I was so relieved to have Steve in the hospital.

I recognized the hospital nephrologist, Dr. Rex Ochi, another well-reputed kidney specialist to whom I refer many of my own patients. He explained that Steve would require emergent dialysis—a kidney machine—and that an internal jugular IV line could be placed in his neck that evening to use for the treatment. There was a whole group of doctors: all of them saw Steve individually; all asked the same set of questions; all expressed surprise and concern at his answers. Steve said later that he thought the young resident looked terrified.

"He thought I was 'CTD,' I bet," said Steve. "I didn't know if he was ready to close the lid on me or what."

Steve was referencing a politically incorrect medical acronym: "circling the drain." Another impolite acronym was "MFC," or "measure for coffin."

Dialysis began the next morning.

Chapter Six

We were old enough—in our mid-fifties—to remember when dialysis was reserved for a special few deemed worthy of the treatment by a Medical Ethics Committee. Steve's childhood pastor had actually chaired that committee, a task so controversial that the pastor's photograph appeared in shadow on the cover of *Life Magazine.*

Dialysis really is a modern miracle, now available to almost anyone who needs it by virtue of technology and Medicare policy. But no matter how miraculous it is, dialysis is a sobering concept.

When I arrived the morning after his admission, Steve was just beginning his dialysis "run." His blood traveled through clear plastic tubing from the exit portal in his neck, filtering through a cylinder of hundreds of micro-filters, winding around the machine's pump mechanism, and finally flowing back to the entry portal in his neck. The treatment took about four hours, with Steve sleeping through most of it.

That evening, his speech still sounded quite bizarre.

"I have encephalipidy!" Steve announced to the nurse who was shaving him.

"*Encehalopathy,* Steve," I corrected. "Can't you tell you're a little nuts?"

"That's what I said," Steve responded indignantly, "encephalipidy!"

I decided to stay at the hospital that night on a rollaway cot.

Steve awoke the next morning to me scratching his back and shoulders. His eyes locked onto an attractive nurse entering the room.

"You are *gorgeous!*" he proclaimed loudly.

"Hey, Steve," I said, "I'm over here. Don't you be talking to another woman with me standing right here! Anyway, it's morning. Are you hungry for some breakfast?"

"Hungry? I could eat a Buick!"

"You'd probably throw that Buick right back up," I said. Steve had been experiencing a fair degree of nausea.

"I'm stoned to the bone! I'm a two-celled mother-fucker!" he announced.

"Steve," I begged, "don't you get it that you are sounding crazy?"

"Okay," he replied, "I probably shouldn't operate a deli meat slicer."

Great. This was just great. My cerebral, uber-witty boyfriend had gone daffy. Futhermore, he looked wild-eyed and disheveled—bearing an uncanny resemblance to Nick Nolte in the mug shot after Nolte's DUI arrest.

Thankfully, Steve's mind did clear, after another round of dialysis and more medical magic. But you really don't know in the middle of it all if your partner will ever be back again.

Dozens of friends called to ask about Steve's condition, particularly after his sister Carole sent out an e-mail with the bulletin. Steve always said that there were two types of friends: the type of friend who will help you move, and the type of friend who will help you move . . . a *body!* I think he heard that in a bar somewhere. Steve collected friends of both varieties. He knew hundreds of people; he remembered the tiniest minutiae of their lives; he nurtured his friendships.

"Body movers" Dick Hagen and Bruce Stanley came to spend time with Steve at the hospital. Dick, now in the commercial real estate business, had met Steve decades earlier. Dick had stopped into Steve's audio store to sell him broadcast advertising time; Steve sold Dick a stereo system instead. Bruce, now an artist and custom audio installer, had owned a competing audio store years ago. Bruce's cartoon illustrating Steve's dialysis experience was hilarious (well, see for yourself on page 41). These wonderful men added precious levity to our precarious situation.

Twelve-year-old Brita saw her dad once in the hospital—or more accurately, once in the hospital on the way to Old Navy. We had given Brita an introduction to kidney disease, but we simply hadn't known that Steve was on such an accelerated track. We layered on bits of information, and Brita was able to see that her dad was alive and looking more normal—or at least less like Nick Nolte.

At Old Navy, Brita and I picked out some new boxer shorts for her dad: a beige pair with black Halloween bats, and a blue pair with moose and bears. It was good to take a little break from the hospital. Although the hospital had been my "home court" for a quarter of a century, it certainly felt different to be on the "other side," to be the recipient rather than the giver of medical care.

Amazingly to us and to the medical staff, Steve's lab numbers began to normalize. He lost an astonishing thirty-five pounds—all fluid. His creatinine fell to 3.0 (healthy is about 1.0). After only two rounds of dialysis, a few days of hospital care with the renal diabetic diet, the kind occupational therapist offering gadgets to help Steve with getting his shoes and socks on, and unanswerable prognostic questions, Steve was ready to go home.

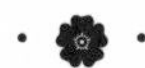

We enjoyed two weeks of apparent redemption before Steve's second descent. I had left the house at 8:15 a.m. By noon, Steve was vomiting uncontrollably. And by late afternoon, he hit the ER again. His creatinine was over 5.0 and his serum bicarbonate had dropped to 15 millimoles/liter. This indicated that Steve was in metabolic acidosis, a dangerous chemical imbalance. All so quickly, and all the result of sudden dehydration in the face of kidney failure.

Dr. Thakur declared that Steve was too unpredictable; he got into trouble too easily. And Steve's wide fluid swings greatly increased his risk of having a heart attack. There was no doubt that he had "End Stage Renal Disease"—treatable only by "renal replacement therapy": permanent kidney dialysis or a kidney transplant.

I called my friend Connie to tap into her medical expertise and, of course, to hear a friendly, familiar voice in the midst of this torture. I hadn't seen this particular set of circumstances in my practice. Neither had Connie, even with her geriatric practice of older, sicker patients—many of whom had diabetes and hypertension. Certainly, she cared for patients on dialysis, but Steve's very precipitous fall into kidney hell was atypical. He was an "outlier," someone who didn't play by the usual rules of medicine.

The whole situation felt surreal to me. Steve was in critical danger; he and I could both feel it. We both knew that our lives would be irretrievably changed by the events of the previous month. We didn't know what to expect exactly, but we understood that there was nothing to do but plod forward. Neophytes in unfamiliar territory, we would follow the expert guidance of those around us—people for whom renal failure was routine.

Because it was time for Steve to begin *permanent* dialysis—possibly for the rest of his life, it was time for Steve and me to go the Northwest Kidney Centers to attend "Kidney School."

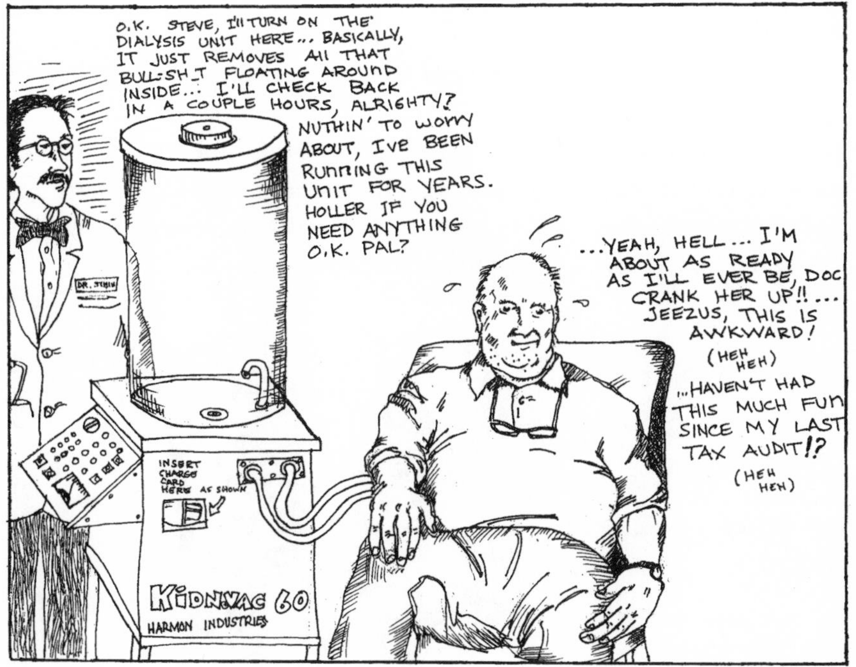

Continued on next page . . .

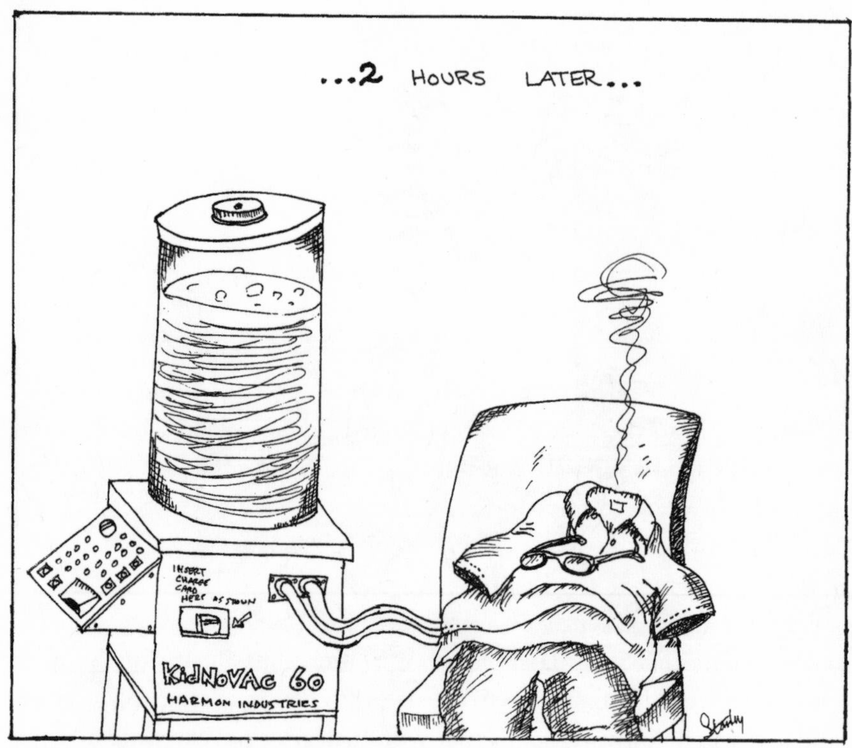
...2 HOURS LATER...
INSERT CHARGE CARD HERE AS SHOWN
KidNoVAc 60
HARMON INDUSTRIES
Stanley

Cartoon by Bruce Stanley, October 2007

Chapter Seven

The Northwest Kidney Centers really must employ the nicest people in the world, extraordinarily kind people who went out of their way to help, to answer questions, to relieve the apparent horror into which we were spiraling. Because of our chaotic work schedules, the very kind social worker, agreed to present a separate "Choices" class for Steve and me alone.

In retrospect, the private lesson was a great idea. It was scheduled on a day when Steve's stomach was "not quite right." That usually meant that Steve would launch—so to speak—into howls of repeated retching, and a series of vomiting spells that would clear out everything down to his duodenum. Kidney School, unfortunately, brought no relief to this pattern. The social worker told me that people didn't usually throw up in her classes. I assured her that it wasn't personal—probably a combination of sick kidneys and diabetic gastroparesis (impared gut motility).

In the Choices class, Steve and I learned about his stark alternatives in addition to a kidney transplant: 1) hemodialysis, where your toxins and extra fluids are filtered out of the blood via a catheter in the neck or a surgically enlarged vein called a fistula, and 2) peritoneal dialysis, where a catheter is placed in the abdomen, and fluid runs in and out of the belly using the peritoneal (gut) membrane as the filter. This seemed terribly ingenious, and apparently was quite adaptable to travel and work demands.

And then, there was the third choice:

"The third choice is to do *no* treatment, and sometimes that is the best option for a person," explained the social worker.

"If a person with End Stage Renal Disease opts for no treatment, *death usually occurs within one to two weeks.*"

Steve and I would come to refer to the third option as "Door Number Three."

Chapter Eight

Brita: what a rich, complex relationship we had, with its brutally tough beginning and its hard-won victories! When I first met nine-year-old Brita, I was genuinely taken by her poise and self-assuredness. Tall and strong with long straight brown hair and multi-colored eyes, Brita greeted me with confidence. We had lunch with her dad at the Nordstrom Men's Grill. Raised in her early years by her dad and his contemporaries—*other* fifty-year-old men, Brita felt fully comfortable ordering a medium rare steak and a Caesar salad.

I remember driving home from that first meeting, flashing involuntarily on the words, "I just met my daughter." I would put that thought away for some time.

Steve and Brita had been a twosome for seven years. There hadn't been other serious relationships since Brita's mom. When Steve helped design his beautiful "architecturally significant" home, Brita's room occupied six hundred square feet—larger than a rental condominium I owned! The den had two adjoining computer stations: one for Brita and one for Steve. Steve invited me to use his computer; but his cats, Triscuit and Oreo, known to me as "the allergens," also shared the desk.

Then, there was the master bedroom. It had no doors, except on the room enclosing the toilet. How could a couple enjoy privacy in this space? Clearly, couplehood had not been considered in Steve's design.

One afternoon in April 2005 and not long after our first luncheon together, I phoned Steve and Brita. It had been an emotional day for me. Several months before, I had decided to end the obstetrical portion of my medical practice, a decision steeped in ambivalence. I loved delivering babies. And while I delivered about fifty babies a year, I had missed only five deliveries in over eighteen years of practice. It was obvious to me that my life needed more balance, and specifically, a life partner. Being on call "twenty-four/seven" was not helping.

"Brita," I said, "I just now delivered my very last baby . . . the last baby I will ever deliver in my whole life!"

"Well, good," she replied, not skipping a beat. "Then, you'll be able to come to the Island and visit me!"

It was a spontaneous, warm comment that soothed my heart at a critical moment. I will always be grateful for her generous response. I didn't realize that I had given up "all those babies" to focus on a new child.

As time went on, however, Brita began to experience some negatives associated with my involvement in her life. I took away much of the time she had previously enjoyed with her dad—alone. I sat in the front seat of the car; Brita was relegated to the back seat. And as a third party, I added a layer of complexity to nearly every interaction. Steve and I could out-vote her, and she began to resist.

At one point, Brita hopped onto her dad's computer and read the e-mails her dad and I had written. In one, I had asked Steve to pick me up after my routine colonoscopy appointment. Pretending to be her dad, *Brita* e-mailed back, indicating that I could *not* be assisted:

"I can't come and pick you up. . . . I would never leave early and not pick up the Bug."

Brita, a.k.a. "the Bug," was busted! A young criminal unmasked! While I was clearly upset, I also recognized this computer "fraud" as serious, sophisticated behavior. Brita was a force of nature, struggling like a little animal to protect the life she knew.

After tightening his computer security, Steve tried to have frank discussions with her and with the three of us together. He and I both emphasized that I wasn't going away. I focused on the truth that nobody could ever take Brita's place in Steve's heart. But it was tough on all of us.

I will never forget the day when this vocal, articulate nine-year-old stared me down in the middle of an intersection and roared, *"I hate every centimeter of you! Get used to it!"*

Every *centimeter*! I was glad to see that Brita was working in the metric system, but horrified that my boyfriend's daughter despised me so vehemently. Part of me wanted to run. But in my heart, I knew that Brita couldn't win—and shouldn't win. Indeed, if she won she lost. Steve and I were growing a loving, interesting relationship. How sad it would be if we all lost out on that? Would Steve resent Brita if I buckled? That was far too much weight to place on this child's shoulders. I stood my ground.

Then I would remember Steve telling me about how Brita, at age four, would lie across the foot of his bed after his near-fatal heart surgery. She had protected him then. Perhaps she had saved him.

I decided to bring out the "big guns"—my twenty-eight-year-old son Tim. He was working as a TV sportscaster in Montana, and was coming to Seattle for a visit. Robust and amiable, Tim could charm anybody. I was certain that Tim could soften Brita.

We decided to have dinner at Tim's favorite restaurant, The Wild Ginger. We didn't know it was Brita's *least* favorite restaurant! When Tim and I arrived, Brita was sitting with her head *on the plate* in front of her. In spite of his heroic efforts, Tim could do nothing to budge Brita out of her miserable isolation. After an excruciating hour, I extended an invitation to bake cookies at my house. Brita refused, and we all left the restaurant.

On the way home, I was nearly in tears. But somehow, Brita's mind changed. Could she still come? Of course. Arriving at my house, Brita ran into my arms. With Cowboy Crunch Cookies baking in the oven, Tim and Brita began to wrestle like well-matched litter-mates! Everybody had fun; everyone was relieved. For Brita, it seemed far better to be included in this "pack."

At the end of a victorious evening, Tim said good-bye to Brita with words from *Rocky*, "Ain't gonna be no rematch, Bug!" Brita and Tim had bonded.

Some time later, Steve, Brita, and I were waiting for a ferry: Steve and I in the front of the VW Touareg, and Brita in the back seat. Suddenly, two nine-year-old feet thrust forward onto the console. Reflexively, I began to massage Brita's feet. Now, so many chapters later, there have been hours of foot massages, dozens of backrubs, and even more "rublets."

I would tuck Brita in at night, naming sheep to the alphabet:

"Agnes," I'd start.

"Barb," Brita continued.

"Cassandra," I offered.

"Dorothy," Brita responded.

"Edna."

And so on, sometimes two alphabets of sheep before Brita drifted off.

There was swimming. And kayaking, school concerts, and rain-soaked soccer games. We rented a dunk tank for Brita's twelve-year-old birthday party: twenty-four squealing pre-teens taking turns pitching a softball at the target and dunking each other in the tank. Tim patrolled the perimeter with water balloons and a Super-Soaker.

These were the sweet intimacies of raising a little girl—a daughter. I had never even thought about raising a daughter before. But this little Brita had landed with both feet on *my* square. Little by little, I came to recognize her as my own.

Chapter Nine

In October 2007—and two days after his second hospitalization for renal failure, Steve and I were returning to Bainbridge Island from an evening blood draw in Seattle. Brita called me on the cell phone.

"Linda, what time are you guys coming home? My stomach hurts." It was a Sunday night—a school night—around eight p.m.

"Where does it hurt, Brita?" I asked.

"In my abdomen."

"Where in your abdomen? Above the belly button or below? On the right side, or on the left? Or all over?"

"Below my belly button, and sort of all over," Brita replied.

"Do you feel like you could throw up?"

"No."

"Can you push on your tummy with your hand, honey? Does it *hurt* when you press on your tummy?"

"Well, sort of—over the lower part."

"Brita, can you jump like a bunny? You know, get up and jump up and down?"

Brita jumped.

"Did it hurt when you landed?" I asked.

"No."

The "jump-like-a-bunny test" was pretty reliable in diagnosing appendicitis, or other acute abdominal mishaps in kids.

"Well, we'll be home by eight, Brita. Don't eat or drink anything, okay? We'll see what you are like when we get home. Okay, honey?"

As soon as we arrived, I examined Brita. She was possibly a little less active than usual for this sturdy twelve-year-old soccer girl. I scratched lightly over the skin of her belly. I rotated her right leg in and out at the hip, and pulled back gently on her right thigh—all maneuvers designed to evoke a response if the appendix is inflamed. Nothing seemed abnormal.

But each time I pressed over "McBurney's Point," in the right lower quadrant of her abdomen, Brita would wince. And attempts to elicit "rebound," i.e. pushing in and releasing the pressure abruptly, consistently produced pain traveling to the right lower quadrant. This looked pretty classic to me for acute appendicitis, and Brita was certainly in the right age group for it.

"I think we better get back to the ferry," I said. "This could be appendicitis, so let's go back over to Seattle and get an evaluation in the ER. If it isn't appendicitis, that's fine. It could just get better on its own, but I think we should go now."

Islanders have to plan their health urgencies around the ferry schedules. Ferries run approximately every fifty minutes, but they stop from 12:55 a.m. to 4:45 a.m. So, you pretty much have to figure out if your situation can wait for several hours, or overnight. There is a way to drive on land around the periphery of Puget Sound, but the trip takes about two hours—treacherous for people in pain. I remember a story of an air ambulance making it to Harborview Hospital in twelve minutes to transport an acute asthmatic, but that was a rare case. While emergency services are reputed to be excellent, I found it ironic that this affluent community seemed so "rural" when it came to medical services.

By the time we got to Swedish ER in Seattle, Brita was looking well, but acted somewhat subdued and still exhibited the same right lower abdominal pain with compression. She was hungry, which didn't fit the typical appendicitis picture in my experience, and she moved without restriction. But she rated the pain as a six on a one-to-ten scale, and she just looked "serious." Women in labor look "serious" when it's the real deal.

A kindly ER pediatrician examined Brita, and her findings were similar to mine. She ordered a blood count, which showed an elevated number of white blood cells—often consistent with infection. She also ordered an ultrasound examination of Brita's abdomen. In an ultrasound exam, sound-conducting jelly is applied to the abdomen and a sound wave probe creates a sonar picture of the underlying structures.

I've seen so many women in pain over my years of delivering babies. I could tell that Brita hurt during the ultrasound exam, especially when the probe explored her right lower abdomen. I showed her how to breathe out when the pressure hurt. Brita tucked her face into the crook of her elbow and just breathed slowly, squeezing my fingers tightly. She never made a sound.

Although the ultrasound study showed that Brita's appendix was slightly enlarged, it wasn't clear enough to make the diagnosis of appendicitis. But the combination of the equivocal ultrasound, the elevated white count, and the reproducible tenderness over the right lower quadrant of the abdomen gave at least a provisional diagnosis of appendicitis. Brita was admitted to the hospital for overnight observation. Steve slept on a rollaway cot. I slept in Brita's hospital bed, my arms around her through the night.

The surgeon examined Brita the next morning: still inconclusive, but requiring observation. There would be no return ferry ride until we had a definitive diagnosis.

By that afternoon, nothing had changed dramatically, except that Brita was now rating the pain slightly higher: a seven-to-eight on a one-to-ten scale. I guess the important point here is that nothing *had* changed dramatically. This is where the surgeon makes a tough call. Nobody wants to take a child to surgery if it's only a false alarm. But the alternative, i.e., waiting until the appendix has ruptured, can be dangerous.

As a resident physician, I remember working on a surgical team when a nine-year-old girl was brought into the ER in full cardiac arrest—

CPR in progress. They even cracked her chest to perform more effective CPR. While this happens several times an episode on TV, it almost never happens in real life, at least not with a nine-year-old child! In the OR, the child's belly was opened: full of pus and a strand-like material called fibrin, all the result of a ruptured appendix. The little girl oozed blood from every IV site. Her heart, beating off and on with the help of medications, finally stopped completely. For the first and only time in my career, I performed open-chest defibrillation: two slender metal paddles with silver dollar surfaces, zapping the little heart into temporary activity. By that time, though, the child's lungs had stiffened—a result of her massive infection. We couldn't close her chest without her heart stopping. All of us around the operating table had young kids of our own. The ongoing code was eventually "called," or ended. I could hear the surgeon sobbing in the bathroom; I cried all the way home.

On Monday afternoon, the decision was made to take Brita to surgery for an appendectomy. With that horrific residency experience as a backdrop, I listened as Brita's anesthesiologist asked her all the routine questions—sprinkled skillfully among inquiries about her soccer team and favorite vacation spots. He started an IV and prepared to transport her to the OR. Steve and I kissed Brita, told her we'd see her when her surgery was completed, and watched as she was wheeled away on the stretcher. As soon as Brita was out of visual range, Steve covered his face with one hand and broke down into quiet sobs; he had never seen his child go through those double doors before. He was still reeling from his own recent hospitalizations, and Brita's vulnerability was too much to bear.

Fortunately, Brita's case was straightforward. The appendix hadn't ruptured, but it was plenty inflamed and needed to come out. She moaned in pain after the surgery. I rubbed her back, stroking her long brown hair through the night, clear that my heart had an opening for a twelve-year-old girl. I had met my daughter after all.

Chapter Ten

Two days after Brita's appendectomy, Steve went to surgery to have a new central line, a large IV catheter, threaded into the internal jugular vein in his neck. He was to begin permanent kidney dialysis the next day.

We had been to the Kidney Center once before for the Choices class or, more correctly, the "No Good Choices" class. Located across from the sprawling not-for-profit Swedish Medical Center with its polished floors and Mark Tobey originals, the little non-profit Kidney Center seemed a bit worn.

The Kidney Center's furnishings were slightly dated; the place ached for a fresh coat of paint and some non-fluorescent lighting. But, as before, what was lacking in décor was well represented in human warmth and compassion—truly, the nicest people on the planet. (It reminded me of my own medical office: there will always be Cheerios ground up in my carpets and plastic dinosaurs strewn across the waiting room floor. But hundreds of magnificent baby photos hang on our walls; and loving, long-term staff members recall each story.)

We came to know three floors at the Kidney Center: the main floor with its reception area, pharmacy, and the Progressive Care Center in the rear; the basement Patient Education Units, dedicated to one-on-one dialysis training; and the sub-basement with its Special Care Unit.

The Progressive Care Unit, where Steve began his In-Center treatments, was a large open room with fifteen Naughahyde recliners for dialysis patients. The chairs had the capacity to assume a variety of positions; most importantly, flat or even tipped head down to remedy severely low blood pressure. Movable carts enabled staff to bring the proper array of syringes, saline flushes for IV lines, bandage supplies, and medications to each patient. I worried about the spread of infection through the unit, even though everyone's sterile technique seemed fastidious. Grimly, each dialysis machine had emergency clamps, a flashlight, and a hand crank attached "so we can give you your blood back if the power goes out."

The nurse began by asking Steve a variety of routine medical history questions. But he also asked, "Are you still working?" and "Did you drive yourself here today?" Steve and I would add our own irreverent questions to the list, like "Are you still feeding yourself?" and "Did you zip your own fly today?"

But it wasn't totally a joke. We would learn that many In-Center dialysis patients did not work; many were on disability. Some patients had lost limbs as a result of diabetes, and others lacked adequate eyesight or dexterity to care for themselves. Some used wheelchairs; many traveled to the Center by Access Bus: publically funded transportation assigned on the basis of medical and financial need. One woman, possibly a homeless woman living in a shelter, brought the apparent totality of her worldly possessions in a shopping cart.

Steve's circumstances were quite different. Until his rapid descent into acute renal failure, he had been working as a consultant in the fitness industry. While he could work from home via computer and telephone, he was required to make occasional business trips from Seattle to Los Angeles, Minneapolis, or Boston. This unusual degree of flexibility was afforded because of his long history as a leader in the industry. He fully intended to continue this work, although the logistics required some clarification at that early point in dialysis.

The woman in the chair next to Steve was easily in her forties. She was watching a Spongebob cartoon on her overhead TV. Some people watched sports; others played computer games; *anything* to help pass the monotonous four-hour time blocks. Steve would usually watch TV, political programs mostly, but often he would simply yield to his growing exhaustion and sleep in the chair.

We could see that In-Center dialysis offered a welcoming refuge for some folks: complete with predictable human interaction, a nutritionist to provide kidney-friendly recipes, and a benevolent financial counselor to help navigate the intricacies of private insurance or Medicare. (Everyone on dialysis qualifies for Medicare by virtue of having End Stage Renal Disease.)

For some, In-Center dialysis could provide a loving structure for a harsh, marginalized life—the problem being, of course, that the admission requirement was kidney failure. For us, however, the In-Center program seemed like a vortex of declining health and disability sucking us irrevocably into its depth.

Every once in a while, it would hit us: "What happened to derail our lives so completely?" or more poignantly, "This is *not* a life we want to live." But there was no way out of this nightmare. Except for some meager choices we *could* make—like the type of dialysis or dialysis schedule—we were stuck. It was heartbreaking, and nothing could be done to change that.

I arrived one evening to pick up Steve after a dialysis run. I had just come from a spinning class, still wearing my baseball cap, T-shirt, cycling tights, and bike shoes with metal clips. The after-hours entrance took me through the Special Care Unit, in the windowless sub-basement of the Kidney Center.

In medicine, the word "special" is often a euphemism. Being medically "special" is like being medically "interesting." It means you're really sick! Your case might be described in a medical journal, but who needs that? Here's a health tip: *Always* strive to be medically *boring!*

The Special Care Unit consisted of rows of dialysis patients in beds, not recliners. These were the sickest of the kidney patients, transported by wheelchairs or gurneys from homes, hospitals, or nursing homes. While they represented the range of ethnicities—kidney disease impacts people of color in disproportionately high numbers—everybody's skin looked sort of a bluish gray. Some people looked as though they could have died weeks before. And, in truth, they all would have been dead had it not been for renal dialysis.

I gathered up Steve and his things, and we headed to the ferry. I reminded myself that Steve, too, would have died over a month before had it not been for dialysis.

(Note: At the time of this writing, the Northwest Kidney Centers was preparing to open a brand new facility: spacious and filled with natural light. The sentence of End Stage Renal Disease, however, remains stark regardless of the facility.)

Chapter Eleven

At the end of October 2007, the Kidney Center sponsored a Kidney Expo held at the Seahawks Stadium Exhibition Hall. It was sort of a trade show featuring "all things kidney." Admission was free, and there were plenty of giveaways and prizes to be raffled.

Bravely trying to embrace our new life, Steve and I headed off to the Kidney Fair. We ran into a few of our new friends: the social worker who taught our Choices class, and the financial counselor. The Center nutritionist was demonstrating a kidney-healthy recipe—shrimp jambalaya, the enticing aroma wafted through the giant hall.

Hundreds of people meandered through the exhibits while we were there, and the fair ran all day long. There were functional but attractive shoes for diabetic feet, cushiony leather recliners for home dialysis, and user-friendly home dialysis machines looking far less intrusive than the In-Center models. Exhibitors gave out candy and gum, little blue rubber kidneys to squeeze to build forearm muscles, and an abundance of literature to read and digest.

Sydney the Kidney, the Center mascot, wandered through the hall. He was flanked by half a dozen happy kids. Sydney stood about seven feet tall: a plump teal blue kidney with mango gym shorts and a mango cap—presumably Sydney's adrenal gland. Steve and I had a Polaroid photo taken with Sydney; we were now officially ensconced in Kidney World.

I was drawn to a booth with the banner, "Traveling with Dialysis." I learned that you could travel by arranging dialysis ahead of time, in kidney centers throughout the world. Then, I spotted the booth of "Dialysis at Sea," a business which coordinated cruise ship travel for dialysis patients and their families. Their vivid brochures outlined an array of destinations: Alaska, the Caribbean, the Mediterranean, and Hawaii. Even China, New Zealand, and Bermuda! Imagine a Christmas cruise aboard a holiday-lit vessel, complete with a board-certified nephrologist and dialysis nurses on board! My life was getting better by the minute.

Then, we met a family practice physician I remembered from decades ago in my training years. It was Dr. Bob Jaffe, the vocal founder of Doctors Ought to Care—or "DOC," a physician-activist organization promoting quit-smoking programs. But here was Dr. Jaffe, sitting in a booth with a dissected cadaver kidney on the table in front of him. He was at the fair to talk about his own personal experience with polycystic kidney

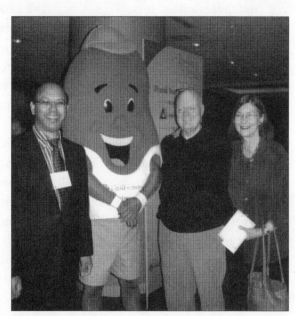

Dr. Smiley Thakur, "Sydney the Kidney," Steve and Linda at a Kidney Fair sponsored by the Northwest Kidney Centers, 2009

disease. Dr. Jaffe had been on kidney dialysis for many years, before receiving a successful kidney transplant. Dr. Jaffe was friendly and candid, and he looked vibrant.

"There's a big difference between being on dialysis and having a transplanted kidney," he said. "Mentally, there was a fog that just lifted right away—as soon as I got my new kidney." He urged Steve to get on the Transplant List as soon as possible.

We met other transplant recipients, too. One had received a kidney that was older than he was! "I'm sixty-five now, but my kidney is going on eighty," he smiled, "and I feel great!"

At another booth, we met a forty-year-old man who could have been a body builder. He wore a muscle shirt; a ropey fistula—an enormous surgically enhanced vein—traversed his beefy right biceps.

"I was on dialysis—as you can see," he said pointing to the fistula, his dialysis-access vein. "And I've always been really active. Skiing, weight lifting—you name it. But things get so much better when you get a transplant."

His eyes locked onto Stephen's eyes. "Get on the list," he said. "You can get a lot of your life back."

I watched Steve closely; something in his face changed ever so slightly. Perhaps it was that these people offered such an active contrast to the very ill people in the Special Care Unit with their prosthetic legs waiting on their wheelchairs. Perhaps it was that Steve was being recruited by these active individuals with whom he longed to identify: "Come join us; your life can be full again."

Steve and I spent a couple of hours at the Kidney Expo. Our outlook was beginning to lift. We were appreciating some new options, some new hope. Perhaps we *could* make this work.

We left the Expo carrying shopping bags of giveaways labeled with the transplant slogan, "Donate Life." As we settled into my Subaru, we waited for the baby blue BMW sports car parked next to us to make its move.

It was the muscle shirt guy with his gnarly biceps, undoubtedly leaving for some grand adventure with his attractive female companion.

Chapter Twelve

In early November 2007, Steve began three-times-a-week dialysis at the Kidney Center's Patient Education Unit. Everyone went through a month of basic training, while receiving dialysis treatments, to ensure they had an understanding of dialysis fundamentals.

Patients like Steve, who elected to perform their dialysis at home, could continue with more intensive training for another four to six weeks in the adjoining Home Dialysis Training Unit. There, the training occurred with daily dialysis treatments, Monday through Friday. Home training candidates had to be capable of reading and grasping an intimidating load of technical information. But they also required adequate vision and a fair degree of manual dexterity. And, the availability of a home helper who could troubleshoot and correct problems if something went wrong with the dialysis—or with the patient.

November was a long month for Steve. Adjusting to wide swings of hydration, Steve would drain as much as four kilograms of fluid—nearly nine pounds—in a session, and leave dialysis looking shrunken. He still carried the extra pounds around his middle, but his eyes would appear sunken in his skull; he looked increasingly debilitated. It would take twelve to twenty-four hours for his system to normalize after a dialysis treatment, or at least to equilibrate to his "new" normal. He felt exhausted. Food started to taste "like minerals," and he ate from memory. In spite of the kindness of the nurses, the four-to-five-hour stints in the Kidney Center basement grew oppressive. The reality of dialysis *forever*—or at least until that new kidney came—hit hard.

Steve desperately wanted to progress to home dialysis, where treatments could be done with David Letterman, where we could capitalize on what Dr. Thakur called "the underwear factor." Being at home meant far more flexibility in scheduling, and no fluorescent lighting.

We learned that there were some clear medical benefits to home dialysis as opposed to In-Center treatments. Home dialysis was usually done five days a week, making the runs shorter. This narrowed the swings in weight and fluid retention. By smoothing out one's chemical balance more effectively, home dialysis afforded greater dietary flexibility also.

There was even a new option: "extended" dialysis, where you got on the machine at bedtime and slept through a slower, gentler six-to-eight-hour run. Slower, more frequent dialysis seemed to replicate real kidney function more closely. Studies had already suggested that "extended" dialysis (referred to us as "nocturnal" dialysis) put less strain on the heart and offered a patient a better quality of life in general. After all, real kidneys work twenty-four hours a day, seven days a week!

As Steve and I began to imagine the logistics of home dialysis, it became apparent that I was going to have to finally move to Bainbridge Island. In early September 2007, Steve and Brita had moved from their beautiful "architecturally significant" home to a lovely cottage in Winery Court, a condominium village within walking distance from the ferry. It was nestled in greenery, and everybody had bedroom doors. I liked the new cottage.

I was already spending most nights on Bainbridge Island anyway, especially from September 2007 when Steve's health became so precarious. But really living on Bainbridge meant diving headlong into the daily ferry commute. It also meant selling my Belltown condo—too expensive to maintain for one to two nights a week. Sadly, the commute would eat up my early morning rowing time.

As we explored the process, Steve and I discussed the idea of marriage.

We had been together for almost three years. I was weary of being the girlfriend, and Steve the consort. Brita needed the stability of a marital unit.

So, on one of our ferry rides to Seattle, and I can't even remember the exact day, Steve asked me to marry him. And I said "Yes."

Steve consulted Brita, who approved. She telephoned me directly.

"Linda, I have a question for you," she said. "Would you be my mom forever?"

"Absolutely," I said. "Absolutely."

I phoned Tim.

"Are you pregnant, Mom?" he asked. We laughed, and he gave his full approval.

Steve asked my mother, also by phone, and she, too, gave her blessing. Our community was gathering around to lend its support.

Steve wanted a party. I would have conducted the ceremony *online* if I could have, with a reception of food samples at the Costco Warehouse. We compromised by planning a tiny family-only wedding at a Hood Canal resort on January twentieth, with a larger party a few months later—"if it took."

Chapter Thirteen

In early December 2007, Steve and I began Home Dialysis Training. We met our two private RN instructors. There was Sarah, a native of Turkey, whose melodious Persian voice could turn any of our mistakes into fortuitous training opportunities. Then, there was Melinda, a petite woman born in the Philippines and raised in Vancouver, BC; she had kids Brita's age, and abundant enthusiasm for our efforts. The nurses would share us with other patients, but the training was virtually one-on-one.

Nives (pronounced "Nee-vus"), the auburn-haired Home Training Director from Venice, Italy, would cruise through the unit to cheer us on—in her designer ensembles and Italian leather boots. Carol and Linda, while not Steve's nurses, were always available, enormously helpful. This group of nurses demonstrated a true esprit d'corps. They obviously loved their work, and the concept that home dialysis could really make a difference in people's lives.

Steve and I would arrive at the Home Dialysis Training Unit every morning, Monday through Friday—shuffling off the 6:20 a.m. ferry. We had our own individual room with a dialysis chair, a whiteboard with specific information relating only to Steve's case, boxes of medical supplies, and a sink. There were four such rooms, clustered around a central nurses' station. But each room *felt* private—a far cry from the open dialysis wards we'd seen.

The particular dialysis machine we used was a NxStage brand machine. It was about the size of a small office copier, and sat on a movable Rubbermaid cart with an IV pole attached. The face of the machine displayed deceptively simple graphics: a green, kidney-shaped button to begin the run, and a red hexagonal stop sign to end it. The dialysis filter and tubing were arranged in a self-contained disposable cartridge. It was truly ingenious medical engineering.

We were given pages of detailed procedural steps. One of us was to read a specific instruction, and the other was to execute the task. In reality, the way this worked was that Steve—sitting in the dialysis recliner wearing his "Jimmy Buffet" shirt—would bark out instructions and then criticize what I was doing.

"Did I *say* it was time to insert the priming spike into the saline bag?" he'd say, fully annoyed. "Don't freelance here, Linda Jo. You're getting ahead!"

And if Steve's criticisms weren't enough, the machine had its own audible alarms: bells with yellow flashing lights for "caution," and bells with red flashing lights for deeper trouble. All of these were backed up, of course, by the realization that if we did do something seriously wrong, Steve's blood could sit in the tubing outside of his body, and clot. A clot in the system could travel to his lungs, and in certain situations, the brain. Furthermore, if I let air into his internal jugular catheter somehow, Steve could have a potentially fatal air embolism—air behaving like a blood clot with equally disastrous results.

We slogged through the training day after day, trying to get Steve's run started by 8:00 a.m. so he'd be a free man by noon. I would leave the center by 9:40 a.m. to run to my own clinic, see my patients, and get home after exercising and charting by 8:00 p.m.

We were adjusting to a new reality: waiting to become proficient enough to graduate from dialysis training, waiting to dialyze at home, and waiting for a new kidney. But, we *were* getting through it.

Christmas and New Years came and went during the training. The best part of the holidays for Steve and me was Tim's new involvement with Brita. On New Year's Eve, Tim and his cousin Michelle supervised Brita, Hannah (Brita's first friend on Bainbridge), and two actual *boys* for a New Year's Eve gathering. Tim and Michelle patrolled the kids, lightly enforcing their rules with kitchen spatulas and duct tape. They kept a written log of behavioral infractions. (For example, "Hannah pees on carpet, 6:30 p.m.," which, of course, was fictional—but fun!)

The Home Training Nurses got wind of our upcoming wedding. "How could you keep this from us?" asked Nives, the director. "We're family!"

And it felt that way; we certainly wanted to take this amazing group of nurses home with us.

In medical school, we learned procedures according to the dictum: "See one, do one, teach one." Dialysis was far too complicated for this training model. In Home Dialysis Training, these patient nurses taught lay people with no medical background whatsoever to execute a complicated sequence of ICU-caliber procedures. People with no prior experience were drawing up their own anticoagulant Heparin, calculating their own dialysis math, i.e., how much fluid to remove from the patient and how long to run the treatment. I thought the whole concept was simply incredible! It made sense, though. After all, nobody cares more about the quality of dialysis than the patient and his or her partner.

Somehow, after weeks of drills, daily practice with the same machine we would take home with us, and several "white knuckle" alarms where the nurses bailed us out of trouble, we were ready to go out on our own. It reminded me a bit of taking a new baby home from the hospital: nobody ever said how complicated *that* process would be!

At the end of our training, all of the nurses came to congratulate us on our achievement. Steve would be their seventieth home dialysis graduate! We received a diploma complete with both of our names, and a gold seal to make it official.

"I feel as proud of this as I did about my MD diploma," I said, stretching the truth only a little.

Steve and I were so grateful. We were grateful for the science and technology that allowed Steve to live, grateful for those innovative thinkers who took renal failure from a death sentence to the alternative of

In-Center treatment, and then to the comfort and flexibility of home. We were grateful that the management of Steve's kidney failure could become part of Steve's routine, not his entire universe. Most of all, we were grateful we'd found each other.

Chapter Fourteen

On January 4, 2008, our graduation day from Home Dialysis Training, Steve and I went out on a real date. Steve's big sister, Carole, had given us tickets to The Jersey Boys for Christmas, and Brita was tucked away with friends on a sleep-over. We took full advantage: a light but elegant dinner at The Crepe de Paris, and a rare evening of musical theater. The show was loud, flashy, and fun; we knew all the music.

Steve and I felt especially close. Hey, let's be fair: we felt triumphant! We had made it through the rigors of Home Dialysis Training, and were ready to go out on our own. Steve and I fell soundly asleep before midnight; it was a well-deserved break.

We awoke late Saturday morning, rested and ready to work. We stopped at the hardware store for storage materials and an emergency flashlight. If the power went off, as it did fairly often on Bainbridge Island, we would have to be able to get Steve's blood back into his body by a procedure called a "manual rinseback." We could do this by flashlight if necessary.

At home, Steve and I unloaded supplies from the VW Touareg: an IV pole, cardboard boxes holding five-liter bags of dialysis solution, and a mechanical fluid warmer. Then, we unloaded the most critical piece—the kidney machine itself—onto our green grocery cart. The machine weighed about seventy-five pounds, and had carrying handles on each side. Somehow, the machine looked less intimidating in the trunk of the SUV. At home, we lugged the machine ever so carefully—one step at a time and with frequent pauses for rest, to the second floor master bedroom, now to be known as the Dialysis Suite.

We assembled our "going on" supplies. We hoisted five of the five-liter plastic bags of dialysis fluid (also called dialysate) onto the IV pole. The bags were connected by individual branches of tubing to the fluid warmer. The arrangement resembled a giant udder, with each bag weighing over ten pounds apiece.

I "set" our work table, actually Steve's nightstand, with a waterproof cover, six twelve cc syringes (two of which I filled with sterile saline), alcohol and iodine packets, strips of tape torn in advance to appropriate lengths, and three packets of four-by-four-inch gauze pads. The waste line, a plastic tube to carry used dialysis flud and excreted liquid—essentially, Steve's new urine—ran along our bedroom carpet and into the bathroom. The waste line was then duct taped to the sink, where the effluent simply ran down the drain.

I drew up 3500 units of the anticoagulant solution, Heparin, into a syringe, and handed Steve the instruction manual. As always, we were to read each step, *never* deviating from the prescribed order.

The routine felt familiar. We had done it so many times in the Home Dialysis Training Unit; we could have done it by memory. Of course, we wouldn't dare "wing it." It was critical to do the procedure exactly right.

We got through the first basic steps: connecting the power cords, connecting the fluid warmer to the kidney machine, and turning on the power. I then inserted the pre-assembled "cartridge" into the machine. The cartridge represented the "guts" of dialysis: pumping blood from Steve's body into a cylinder containing zillions of tiny microfilters, all compacted into what looked much like an oil filter. In the cylinder, Steve's blood was allowed to interface with the dialysis fluid by way of the filter membranes. "Bad" or toxic molecules and excess fluid would move *out* of Steve's blood by crossing the membrane. Certain "good" molecules from the dialysate would move through the filter membranes *into* Steve's blood. It is important to understand that the blood itself never actually mixes with the solution. I think it is easiest to think of the filter as a semi-permeable wall with blood on one side, and dialysis fluid on the other side—and molecules meandering across the membrane to achieve the correct chemical balance. It is also helpful to remember, should anyone find this daunting, that this *is* Nobel Prize-winning medicine!

By pressing the cartridge into the kidney machine at specific anchors, we activated sensors which, in turn, engaged critical alarms to signal when blood flow had stopped, clotted, or when air had entered the system. The five giant IV bags were then connected by another tubing system to the fluid warmer, which then fed the fluid into the kidney machine itself.

Steve and I watched the machine's graphic screen scroll through its various settings, its inner computer preparing for the dialysis run. Then, as we had done so many times before, we programmed in the specific amount of fluid to be withdrawn from Steve's blood—essentially, the body fluid he was unable to excrete by making urine. In Steve's case, twenty-five liters of dialysis fluid was used to *clean* the blood, but only about one or two liters of fluid would be actually removed from his blood. This was the equivalent of making approximately one or two quarts of urine! We then programmed the rate of blood flow for the treatment, in his case 400 milliliters, almost a pint, of blood per minute. Roughly seventy-five *liters* of blood would be circulated through the kidney machine in the entire run!

I put on my latex exam gloves, and Steve and I both donned surgical masks.

"Are you ready?" I asked.

"It's a go, captain," he said.

With all my supplies within reach, I took hold of the "arterial port" of Steve's internal jugular catheter. The nomenclature is confusing because there was really only *one* internal IV line housing two connection ports. The arterial port led blood away from the body; the venous port led blood back to the body.

"Breathe in," I instructed as I removed the cap from the arterial port of the central line.

Steve obeyed. If he didn't hold his breath at this point, air could be sucked into the system, creating a dangerous air embolism.

I attached an empty syringe.

"Breathe out," I pulled back on the syringe, drawing blood out of the arterial port.

"Thank God," I said. "That was easy."

Switching syringes, and attaching one filled with saline, I squirted the blood-filled syringe onto a gauze pad.

"No clots!" I cheered.

I pushed the saline into Steve's central catheter.

"Breathe in," I instructed, as I removed the cap from the venous port and attached a Heparin-filled syringe. The process was repeated on the "venous" portal. Again, no clots. I then connected the plastic tubing from the kidney machine to the central line ports—the tubes that would carry Steve's blood to and from the machine. We were off to a good start, and we both started to relax.

"Okay," said Steve, "let's run through the checklist." Melinda had compared this final checklist to the procedure used by a 747 pilot preparing for take-off.

"Blood lines connected to the catheter ports?" Steve asked.

"Yes," I responded.

"Catheter clamps open, arterial and venous?"

"Check."

"Fluid warmer bag filled? Warmer outlet connected to the machine with clamps open?"

I nodded.

"Waste line connected, and unclamped?"

"Yes."

"All volumes and flow rates programmed in?"

"Got that."

Steve paused and took a deep breath.

"Hit the kidney!" he commanded.

Reflexively, I punched the little green kidney-shaped button. We were "on," watching with a mix of relief and amazement as blood flowed from Steve's body into the machine, through the filter, and back to his body. We diligently recorded Steve's vital signs and pressure readings from the machine. I adjusted the blood flow rate to its maximum, with the machine cranking louder in response.

So far, so good: no alarms! We had, of course, about three hours and fifteen minutes yet to go at that point.

Steve's sister Carole had come to the Island to help with this all-important maiden voyage. Carole was not only a "body mover," as Steve would say, she would *look* for a body to move for you!

Carole was ten years Steve's senior, but she seemed younger than both of us in her energy and activity level. She had hit the ground running, starting her family at age sixteen, with three daughters and a son by age twenty-five. After a divorce, Carole went back to college for a business degree. She told me once—while we were kayaking—that she had wanted a job with the "three T's": travel, technology, and trucks. She found that in an international position with Paccar. Carole knew no limits. At fifty and with no prior experience, Carole "auditioned" to crew a five-woman sailboat traveling from San Francisco to Hawaii. She was accepted, and completed the voyage without a hitch. After her kids had grown, Carole moved to an upscale one-bedroom condo near the Pike Place Market. She was willing to help any of her kids, her nine grandchildren, or four great-grandchildren at a moment's notice, but she didn't want the whole crew descending on her at once—or moving back! Such limits are easier to enforce with a smaller space. Carole maintained her physical fitness through Volksmarching and water aerobics. She did volunteer stints at the USO, and worked for "play money" at the Children's Hospital Catering Department. Carole had even taken Brita, at age eleven, to Norway for a three-week adventure. She was an inspirational woman by any standard.

Carole and I sprung into action once Steve was on his dialysis run, organizing shelves and sorting through boxes of equipment from the Kidney Center. The sixty cardboard boxes from NxStage hadn't come yet, but we had to make space for them in our blessedly large bedroom.

Carole and I joked that we might leave and go out shopping for a bit; clearly that wasn't an option. Dr. Thakur had said that Home Dialysis was sort of like boiling potatoes on the stove. You could do other things, but you had to be within earshot in case your potatoes boiled over.

As Steve's dialysis run ground to a close, we read through our instructions once again. I rechecked my "going off" supplies: Heparin flushes and sterile caps for the catheter ports. We both put on our surgical masks again.

I disconnected Steve's arterial line from the catheter port in his neck, and placed a new sterile end-cap on the port. Then, I turned to disconnect the venous line.

It wouldn't budge! I tried and tried, with every ounce of strength I had—no progress! I even had Steve try, but be couldn't get the connection to budge either.

We were in trouble. We couldn't leave Steve connected to the machine; his blood would clot within minutes. And the 1-800 Helpline was out of the question!

Steve glared at me from behind the mask, looking as though I was plotting to murder him. The hemostats, delicate but sturdy surgical pliers, hadn't been included in our supplies! And neither of us had noticed.

"Pliers!" shouted Steve. "Carole, get the pliers from the toolbox!"

Carole ran downstairs as Steve and I struggled on, trying desperately to disconnect the line. Carole bounded back, carrying household pliers and a small set of needle nose pliers.

"Will these work?" she asked.

They weren't sterile, and we didn't care. I clamped the two sets of pliers onto Steve's delicate catheter connection and twisted hard in opposite directions. It worked!

"Thank heaven!" I proclaimed with relief.

"Now I'll probably get a catheter infection," moped Steve—irritated but relieved.

"Yes, and it'll be my fault!"

We finished the treatment and all went to Casa Rojas for Mexican dinner; the three of us were exhausted.

After dinner, Steve and I started what was to become a ritual: going over the evening's run and reviewing what we'd learned from it.

I had been wounded by Steve's glare. But he was just scared and who could have blamed him? Carole pointed out that our problem was simply mechanical; with the proper set of hemostats, we could easily avoid this problem in the future.

In a nutshell, our first tenuous run allowed us to invent the "Dialysis Serenity Prayer":

God grant us the strength to even start this dialysis run,

The courage to troubleshoot and correct the problems we encounter,

And the wisdom to work as a team *without antagonizing the woman who's managing your jugular!*

Chapter Fifteen

With our wedding coming up on January twentieth, Steve and I took Brita and two of her "girly-girl" friends for an overnight at the Alderbrook Resort on Hood Canal. We had two agenda items: first, to check out the facility for our mini-wedding ceremony, and more importantly, to meet with Steve's cousin, Don Cornell, the Lutheran pastor who was to marry us.

We set out with the three twelve-year-olds to meet Don and his wife JoAnn at their log home, minutes from the resort. I had met Don once before at a family gathering: a kindly man in his seventies with a long history of pastoring all over the world, mostly in the Middle East. JoAnn was the quintessential grandmother—offering the girls TV, video games, and extra snow clothing to play outside. The girls vacated happily to the wintery yard, and the four adults assembled around the enormous dining room table.

Don and JoAnn's home reflected much about them. It was a log home—not a cabin, but a full-sized home. Their furniture was expansive and inviting, an eclectic mix of Ethan Allen and the Middle East. Cozy woven upholstery blended with sleek brick leather. It all worked to produce an inviting atmosphere where folks could gather and feel welcomed.

Don and JoAnn shared the story of their *own* wedding. Their honeymoon had been at Alderbrook, fifty years before!

"I'll see if Mother can find the picture of young Steve catching JoAnn's bridal bouquet," he smiled. Steve had attended Don and JoAnn's wedding at age eight.

Don eased into the details of the wedding ceremony. We wanted our union to be official. Neither of us was particularly religious, but we both considered ourselves to be moral, spiritual folks.

"So, how did you two meet?" asked Don.

"Oh, we went to high school together, to Queen Anne," said Steve, referring to the 1906 institution, since converted into pricey condominiums.

"No kidding!" replied Don.

"We didn't even *know* each other in high school, Don," I said.

"We met over coffee three years ago," explained Steve. "We ran in totally different circles in high school—representing the extremes of the academic spectrum. I'm sure Linda Jo's parents wouldn't have let me in the house."

He might have been right about that point. Steve had been a bit of a hoodlum in high school. No serious trouble, but plenty of mischief. He had a scrapbook full of pictures of his high school buddies, usually holding bottles of beer. Then, there was a clipping from the *Magnolia News* describing Halloween antics where Steve and his friends lit car tires on fire and rolled them down the steepest hill in the neighborhood.

"Come on, Steve," I said. "Let's be complete. We met online—you know, on Match.com. I wrote an ad with the heading, *"I'd like to meet a nice Democrat."*

Don and JoAnn both laughed, both Democrats.

"Yes," Steve said, "and I responded right away with 'Kerry delegate here!'"

Steve hadn't quite come to terms with Internet dating; the idea still made him squirm a little.

"Listen, Steve," I said, "I know you don't always share this information, but this is how people meet these days. Where do you meet people after college anyway?

"Besides," I explained to Don and JoAnn, "it cuts through all the nonsense. You know at a glance who drinks, who smokes—who has a dog! You know: the basics! It's efficient, that's all."

Steve sighed as I told the rest of the story. As we talked about our relationship, it was abundantly clear to all off us what Steve and I saw in each other. We were both complicated people, with complicated lives. We were both irreverent in our humor and passionate about our politics. Our moral values were synchronous; we reinforced each other's non-negotiable sense of doing the right thing. We were practical and creative, and even more importantly, we were comfortable just *being* with each other. Perhaps it was our shared culture: our parallel early lives which provided a common template of security, a sense of just "coming home" when I was with him. Perhaps it was that we were so similar in our independence that we both identified ourselves as "unemployable" by other people. We recognized that we were both "acquired tastes," as Steve would say, "not everybody's cup of tea." But we were a great match for each other, verified over and over again by the life events that had tested our mettle.

Don and JoAnn just smiled knowingly through it all. We worked through the details of our wedding ceremony as my new little girl and her friends played outside in the snow.

CHAPTER SIXTEEN

By mid January 2008, Steve and I had made it through eight or ten home dialysis treatments. We were starting to feel marginally competent or, at least, not as terrified that something catastrophic would happen. We had experienced a few yellow and red alarms, and we had been able to troubleshoot and manage the problems that occurred.

We arranged our physical surroundings as efficiently as possible: our spacious, woodsy bedroom with a view of a natural ravine and man-made stream was now overtaken by sixty cardboard boxes containing dialysis fluid. Collectively, these created a footprint of four feet by ten feet, and stood about four feet high. A separate alcove housed an eight-foot bookcase of medical supplies, and there was yet another nook with more cardboard boxes. Thankfully, we had the space for all of these supplies. We imagined this "stuff" landing into someone's one bedroom apartment—like Jeff's, for example.

Our home dialysis suite featured an excessive one-hundred-twenty-inch projector screen for watching TV. Actually, with Steve in the business of home electronics, he got the screen for under two hundred dollars, and his friend Bruce installed the monstrosity at no charge. It was great—I mean, who could complain? It just seemed so excessive. Steve clarified that it was a "guy thing." Dialysis with David Letterman;

indeed, we could practically see David's pores!

So our physical setup was as good as it could possibly be. But a bedroom with a dialysis machine can seem more like an ICU room than a bedroom—clearly unromantic. As if romance was an issue! There we were, just days from our planned wedding and Steve and I began to bicker.

The dialysis schedule was taking a physical toll on me. After all, *my* little day job—running that *medical* practice—was fully occupying in itself. Plus, I was trying desperately to get to two spin classes and two weight-training sessions per week; the bare minimum I could do to maintain my hard-won physical fitness. The commute to Bainbridge Island added a minimum of two hours to my day. I would arrive home at eight p.m., physically exhausted and emotionally spent, with four hours of dialysis stretching on ahead.

I started to fray, and Steve didn't get it! I was weary to my bone marrow. My body hurt. I resented Steve's expectations. One evening I missed the 7:20 p.m. ferry by three minutes while waiting for a freight train to pass. I was later than usual because I had stopped at my Belltown condo to check on some financial records; with all our dialysis activities, I'd missed my estimated tax deadline, something I'd never do under normal circumstances.

Steve lit into me the next morning. "You either live here or you live in Belltown!" he bellowed. "There is no reason you can't bring your ledgers here and use this computer!"

"I hate your computer, Steve," I blasted back. "It's too slow and it doesn't work like mine. Besides, that's not the issue!"

With two days until our wedding, I stormed off to catch the morning ferry, exhausted and furious. He could dialyze in the basement of the fucking Kidney Center—the Seventh Layer of Dante's Inferno! It would be fine with me! He didn't get for one minute the sacrifice I was making, the sacrifice he was imposing on me. I resented him deeply.

I was especially frustrated because Barb, my office manager, had proposed a perfectly logical plan whereby Steve could dialyze in my medical office. Our physical plant would be ideal. We had a private exam room which could be designated exclusively for his treatments;

we had the storage capacity. Steve could set up his phone and laptop, and do his work while dialyzing. We even had an alarm bell. Steve could call for help if he ran into a medical problem—or if his pillow needed fluffing!

The problem was this: it would be an inconvenience to *Steve!* He would have to make the daily ferry commute, the commute *he* said was no problem!

I phoned Nives at the Kidney Center to see if it would be permissible to dialyze Steve in my medical office. He would be my husband in another two days, after all, unless one of us self-combusted—or walked out!

"Yes," said Nives, "You can dialyze at work. You can do it in an RV. You can dialyze on a boat. I don't care."

Our basic goal, besides the new kidney, of course, was to start doing "extended" dialysis overnight at home. We could both sleep through the treatments in our big bed with a bedwetting alarm under Steve's arm in case his IV lines became disconnected.

If Steve would just cooperate, we could do February treatments in my office. We'd take the kidney machine to Steve's important trade show in San Diego in early March, and return to start training on "extended" dialysis or, as Nives would say, "The Cadillac of Dialysis."

I approached Barb. Barb is one of the kindest, most precious people I've ever known. She had worked with me for over twelve years, and in that time, I'd observed that Barb could talk to anybody about absolutely anything. Tough subjects? No matter. Once, I convinced Barb that it was within her job scope to tackle a particularly troublesome flatulence problem with one of our former staff members. Barb did it with characteristic grace and dignity.

"Linda," said Barb, "Steve doesn't make decisions as fast as you do. But here, you need to give him the facts and tell him exactly what you need. Send him an e-mail, and spell it out."

Steve respected Barb, always saying that Barb was so effective in managing people because she was good with big dogs—like German shepherds. Barb could distill everything down to a matter of "pack psychology," and she was usually right.

I e-mailed my groom:

Dear Steve,

I am writing out of deep concern for you and your dialysis arrangements. Our lives are very complicated right now, and probably always will be. With a two-hour daily commute and now a four-hour dialysis run after my intense workday, I am not sure I can continue!

I appreciate that you are the one with the kidney disease, and for that I am truly sorry. But I am the one whose schedule is taking the present impact. Please remember that I am now taking every Tuesday off from work to facilitate your multiple medical appointments. I have cancelled my own patient appointments to be with you in the hospital or at critical appointments. I earnestly want to help you. I want nothing more than for you to live well; for that matter, for you to live at all! These are the stakes, and they are very high!

So, very clearly, I cannot continue to run a full-time medical practice, commute to Bainbridge, and do evening dialysis. I look forward to overnight dialysis. To continue doing your daily treatments, I offer you treatments in my office. *We will provide a dedicated room—complete with phone and computer outlet. You may bring your laptop and a TV; we have a call bell for emergencies.*

We can commute on the same ferry, and get your treatments done by noon. You have always said that the commute is less of a problem for you.

I will be able to complete my medical charting, dictation, and maybe even see more patients without the present time crunch.

I will continue to serve as your dialysis helper until you get that new kidney. I do not think we can afford to hire a dialysis technician for home, but that would be another option. Please consider these points, Steve. I have tried to help; now please try to help me.

Love, Linda Jo

Steve e-mailed back:

> *My dearest Linda Jo,*
>
> *I fully understand that this is more than you committed to, or forecasted on the front end. It has taken us both by surprise. The time and logistics are more difficult than we had thought, and overnight dialysis is still an unknown. However, I hope it still represents the most promise, pre-transplant. I am willing to work with you and your program . . . ferry, parking fees, and whatever comes with doing dialysis at your office. It is surely a mixed blessing/gift. Let's talk logistics soon, as I have to order supplies ASAP.*
>
> *I will ask that you consider some alteration to* your *Seattle-based activities, and look for ways to integrate yourself into the Island activities. Quality personal training and cycling classes are available on the Island.*
>
> *I need you, and Brita needs you to be happy and present in our lives and in the home that we share. The chaos of the past few months should be easing up a bit, and the need for your Tuesday services declining.*
>
> *The planning scope should be larger than just the kidney. How we live, play, and work needs careful review. I want this set of conditions to work for you, as best they can.*
>
> *Love, Steve*

Steve's letter and the biting conversation that followed inflamed my raw little nerves even more. So now I was to spin on Bainbridge, do my strength training on Bainbridge, and get on the earliest possible boat home. Would he be asking me to leave or move my medical practice next?

We had an icy, rugged evening. I completed Steve's dialysis run, barely speaking to him, but handling his central line with meticulous care.

Steve was in a position of singular vulnerability. But I had to take care of myself, too! If I couldn't work and couldn't play, at least a little, I'd be of no use to anyone. We communicated minimally, neither of us wanting to "poke a skunk."

Our wedding was coming up in two days!

Chapter Seventeen

Saturday, January 19, 2008, was my mother's ninetieth birthday. My mom had been a homemaker, devoting her time to my sister Bonnie and me, and to my father until his death just after their fiftieth wedding anniversary. My mother was an extremely bright woman, having earned a Master's degree in speech pathology at the University of Michigan at a time when few women went to college at all.

My mom lived alone in her little Magnolia home—in a lovely Seattle neighborhood—in the home where Bonnie and I grew up. After my dad died of a massive stroke in 1991, Mom wanted to continue to live in the same home. It was her security; she had her garden, her familiar things. Best of all, she could manage independently as long as a few of us provided minimal services to assist her. My sister took her shopping once a week. Tim had begun weekly movie nights, bringing Grandma an assortment of World War II era films, musicals, and the like. Sometimes, my niece Michelle would join them.

My mom had a long-term arrangement with her hair dresser and former neighbor, Randi. Randi would pick up Mom every Monday morning and drive her to the beauty shop to style her hair. I'd pick her up when she was finished, and drive her home.

"Do anything you want with my schedule," I told my staff, "but don't even think of messing with my mom's shampoo and set!"

Bonnie and I would help Mom with banking, medications, and dental appointments. Mom had finally acquiesced to wearing a "Lifeline" alarm necklace. She hadn't had to activate the alarm, but the fact that she wore it was reassuring to the family. I'd call her every night to do a "Life Check," just making sure that she was okay.

Sometimes, my mom gave me advice—beyond her standard: "Just get *up* every day!" For example, she would say, "Linda, you do too much," or "Why don't you wait and marry Steve when he's healthier?"

Steve's health was difficult for Mom to grasp. Small wonder: here she was at ninety with no major health issues. Steve, at fifty-eight, grappled with the reality that better health was a full kidney transplant away. Were there other subtexts to my mom's question? Aren't there *always* subtexts to a mother's questions? Certainly, I knew that my mom wanted the best for me; she worried that I might be moving headlong into a life of increasing hardship. Perhaps she worried that I would be widowed, or shouldered with the responsibility of raising a teenaged daughter alone. Long ago, I remember my mother's "curse" at a time of her frustration with my *own* vocal teenaged behaviors: "I hope when you grow up you have a daughter *just like you*!" she said. Perhaps she worried that that curse had come true.

Mom shared her birthday parties with Bonnie's son Michael, delivered at home twenty-four years earlier, courtesy of the paramedics. Michael, a University of Washington English literature graduate, recorded his own music and earned his rent cooking at The Honey Hole. Mike had suggested a favorite vegetarian restaurant for our celebration.

So, Mom, Bonnie and her husband Alan, Michelle, Michael, Tim, Brita, Carole, Steve, and I all met at Café Flora for a sweet, relaxed birthday brunch. It was pleasant and easy, just enough of an event to confer the appropriate honor, but not so much as to feel overwhelming.

After brunch, Steve, Brita, and I stopped at REI to buy some new snowboard gear for Brita. She had been invited to go with a friend on their family outing to Jackson Hole the week after the wedding—far too great an opportunity to miss.

Steve and I ended the day—the one before our wedding—with dialysis.

Was our situation ideal? Hardly!

Was my fiancé with his history of heart surgery, diabetes, End Stage Renal Disease and now home dialysis a "trophy husband?"

Well, he was certainly not perfect. But I'd never found a man as witty, as interesting, or as comfortable as Steve Williams. And there was nobody who knew *me,* and loved *me*—all idiosyncrasies disclosed—as Steve Williams did. Possibly—just possibly, Steve was the perfect match *for me.*

Chapter Eighteen

Our wedding was scheduled for 3:30 pm. Sunday, January 20, 2008 at the Alderbrook Resort on Hood Canal. It was a glorious setting: a broad expanse of deep blue water flanked by crystalline mountains. The Resort sprawled around a massive Northwest lodge, near the estates of the Gates and Nordstrom families. It was easy to appreciate how families had frequented the resort for generations of summer vacations and special events.

Steve, Brita, and I set out for Alderbrook, stopping first at the Town and County Market in Winslow to pick up our wedding cake. We had selected a simple chocolate layer cake with white butter cream frosting, decorated with the names, "Linda, Steve, Brita, and Tim." It was beautifully done: yellow flowers with yellow and green trim.

"Do you like it, Brita?" I asked.

"Yes, I do like it," she answered. "My name's bigger than Tim's!"

"Peace in the valley," I noted to Steve. "Could we swing by the Bainbridge Bakers to see if Scruffy Bob's there?"

Bob Ness, or "Scruffy Bob," as we knew him was a third-generation Bainbridge Islander and somewhat of an Island fixture. He worked in computers, designing web pages, and he produced video training and marketing materials. He had also written a screenplay and was awaiting its acceptance by the film industry. Scruffy was highly active in Alcoholics Anonymous—clean and sober for decades. Bob had generously sponsored countless Islanders through their transitions into sobriety.

I had met Scruffy Bob at the Career Corner, morning coffee at the Bainbridge Bakers, where Bob, Steve, and a random crew of other unshaven, but good-hearted souls would commiserate about the working world. They'd sit and sip, watching Islanders in business suits pick up their lattes-to-go on their way to the Seattle ferry. On their way to a "J-O-B," as Bob would say. Being committed to my work, but unemployable by *others*, I qualified as an "honorary member."

The group would chat about other issues besides work: politics, conflict resolution, and raising teenagers. Tom Martin, a web designer with a fresh hip replacement, would tell stories of raising his own kids: like meeting his daughter's new boyfriend while cleaning surgical instruments in his front yard. Tom thought butchering a sheep while meeting a daughter's new boyfriend sent an unequivocal message of parental love. The group was joined periodically by a family law attorney, a writer, and even our own Soundgarden rock star, Ben Shepherd. I googled him up and learned that he was kind of a hellion on stage, spitting on the crowd—or so they said. But at the Career Corner, Ben was a thoughtful and generous man who was eloquent in discussing political matters. Lively discussions, always!

The Career Corner repeatedly proved its support for our family. Bob's commitment to Steve was solid; he told me he was good for a kidney if he matched Steve, and he meant it.

We drove into the bakery parking lot. Bob was there in his corduroy jacket and multi-colored knit cap; shaving had been optional, and Bob had opted out.

"So have you done it yet?" he asked, smiling broadly.

"We're on our way," said Steve.

"Well, good for you!" Bob said to Steve.

Bob turned to me, shaking his head. "And as for you . . . what the *hell* were you thinking?"

We had been blessed by Scruffy Bob. Steve, Brita, and I headed up the highway to Alderbrook.

We couldn't have ordered a more beautiful day for our wedding. January twentieth was crisp and clear. As my dad used to say, "The mountains were out!"

Alderbrook was a special place for many of us. Certainly, it was magical for Don and JoAnn, who had honeymooned there fifty years before. Steve's father, who died at only fifty-six of congestive heart failure and probably diabetes, had been a stonemason. He had commuted daily from Seattle to Alderbrook to lay the stone for the massive fireplace in the original Alderbrook Lodge; Steve was just a boy at the time.

For Steve and Brita and me, it was one of the first places we remembered having genuine fun as a family. During our first trip to Alderbrook, Brita and I played "fish games" in the swimming pool. That was also the trip where Brita and I taught Steve to recite the whimsical names of the TV characters, the Teletubbies, and he would do so over and over again, provoking unstoppable giggles from Brita.

Brita helped me get dressed for the wedding, straightening my already-straight brown hair with a special iron. Our dress code was "business casual." Brita begged me not to wear my usual black: "You're too Goth, Linda!" I wore a new "hot fudge" outfit from Chico's—nothing too dressy, but at least something new. Steve wore a dark blue business suit, and looked as elegant as one *can* look, missing a tooth. (He'd had an extraction following a recent abscess, and was in the process of maturing a titanium implant.) I'm pretty sure Steve bribed Brita not to wear jeans; she looked grown up and beautiful in a gray sweater and skirt.

We met Don and JoAnn in the enormous woodsy lobby of the resort. Bonnie, Alan, Michelle, Tim, Carole, and my mom were all there, all excited. Michael had to work, but he had given us his good wishes the day before. We made our way to the cozy library, the room designated for our ceremony.

Steve and I—*and* Brita and Tim—stood before Don, in front of the rest of our group, everyone seated in comfortable leather chairs around the fireplace.

Tim and Brita served as our ring-bearers and our witnesses. The rings—simple, wide Titanium bands—each hid specific engravings.

Mine read "Stephen – Mom – Timanoo – Brita." Steve's read "Lindajo – Dad – Britabug – Timmer." The engravings defined our new family, each ring containing the sweet names Steve and I had given our biological children so many years before.

I glanced around the room. My mom looked a little misty. Tim and Brita were beaming at each other, and everyone else watched expectantly, poised to take pictures.

The ceremony was simple. Steve and I had gone through it the week before. Neither of us was able to get through the vows without breaking down. He did better than I did at the actual ceremony. I cried, but at least the crying wasn't out of control.

"I take you Stephen," I repeated,

"To be my husband from this day forward.

To join with you and share all that is to come.

I promise to be faithful to you until death parts us."

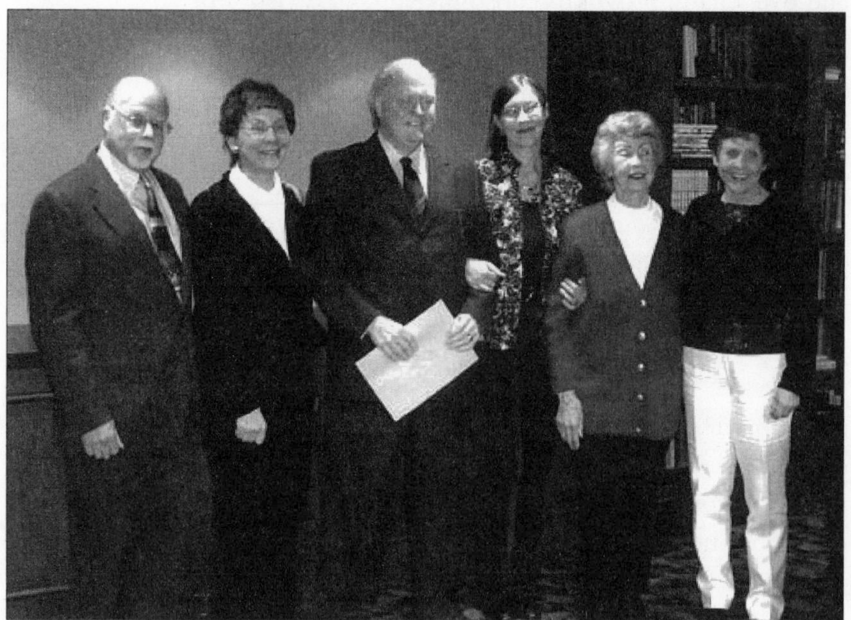

Alan Mearns, Bonnie Mearns (Linda's sister), Steve, Linda, Florence Gromko (Bonnie and Linda's mom—at ninety!), and Steve's sister Carole Williams gather after the wedding at Alderbrook Resort on Hood Canal

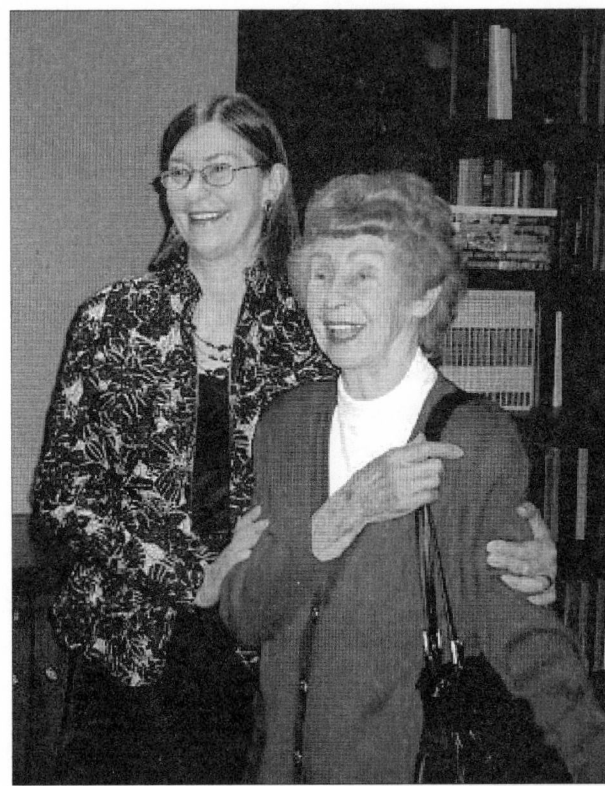

Linda and her mom at the wedding

To join with you and share all that is to come! I wondered briefly what that might mean. Here we were in our mid to late fifties: Steve on dialysis with a central IV line in his jugular vein, a son still finding himself, and a daughter perched on the brink of adolescence.

But it was time for photos and food. We had a simple sit-down dinner in the adjoining wine room, and the charming little wedding cake decorated with the names of our new family. After dinner and toasting, Bonnie and Alan took Mom back to Seattle by ferry. The rest of us settled in at Alderbrook for the night.

Michelle and Brita shared one luxurious hotel room, and Tim had another room to himself. They were all up for hours into the night, with Michelle and Brita swimming until the pool closed. Later the three "kids," ages twelve, twenty-seven, and thirty-one, took off to forage for food. Everything was closed at the resort, so they found a Texaco station and convenience store at the nearby Skokomish Indian reservation. Twenty-seven dollars covered a feast of pure junk: seventeen items including beef stick and ranch dressing, Pringles, Cheetos, popcorn, and candy—all of the essentials!

The next morning, the early risers joined for breakfast before Michelle and Tim had to return to Seattle. Then, the remaining women—Carole, JoAnn, Brita, and I—met at the fabulous Alderbrook Spa for massage treatments.

A permission waiver was required for Brita's facial.

"Are you her mom?" the receptionist asked.

"Yes," Brita and I answered in concert.

We dressed in our Turkish towel robes and spa sandals, absorbing the herbal aromas and soft music around us. Then, we separated for our individual massage treatments.

Steve found us afterwards in the Relaxation Room, looking a bit out of place in his jeans and outdoor jacket. The four of us women sipped hot tea, still in our fluffy robes—candles flickering, lulling music in the background. It was a wonderful event, start to finish.

But, my Cinderella coach was soon to turn into a pumpkin. We reminded ourselves of Steve's short tether, and headed back to Bainbridge Island for the day's dialysis run.

Chapter Nineteen

On Wednesday, January 23rd, freshly married, Steve and I attended the Kidney Transplant Class at the University of Washington. This was an important milestone for us, the first step on the way to getting that new kidney—that new way of life.

I had already submitted my application to be Steve's kidney donor. I had had my initial physical examination, and had blood drawn for basic chemistry tests, and for blood typing. A questionnaire probed my reasons for wanting to donate my kidney. The answers seemed obvious to me: I was interested in having a *living* husband, and twelve-year-old Brita needed a set of two healthy parents.

If, by some miracle, Steve and I "matched," I would have one of my kidneys removed through a small incision over my pubic bone. The process, assisted by laparoscopy, the keyhole and video camera surgery, would require a few days in the hospital and a couple of weeks' recovery time.

Steve's surgery would be more complicated. The surgeon would implant my healthy kidney into Steve's pelvis, leaving his two unhealthy kidneys untouched. We would undergo the surgeries simultaneously, so that my kidney could go directly into Steve with no "down time." A living, matched kidney would promise Steve the best possible results. The risks to me would be small, though certainly present, as in any surgery. The catch for me would be that if my remaining kidney failed or was somehow injured, I too would travel down the path of renal failure. By this time, I felt I had a fair measure of informed consent. I knew intimately the reality of dialysis and the declining health leading up to it.

The obstacles for the transplant loomed ahead:

1) Would my blood *type* be compatible with Steve's? (Steve had type A blood, so he would need a donor of types A or O.)
2) Would Steve's blood have antibodies that would mingle adversely with proteins in my blood?
3) Would Steve be *healthy* enough to receive a transplant? His pre-operative evaluation would almost certainly include a cardiac catheterization to ascertain whether or not he would need another heart bypass surgery. Dr. Thakur said that it was not uncommon for diabetic patients to require some form of cardiac intervention—an angioplasty and stent, or bypass, perhaps—before getting a new kidney.
4) Finally, was my *own* kidney function strong enough to allow me to live healthfully with only one kidney? You can live well with only one kidney, but not if it's second rate.

We learned that if we did not match each other but were good candidates in other respects, we might participate in a "couples match." We'd be matched with another couple in the same predicament. I'd give my kidney to the other couple's kidney patient; their healthy spouse would give his or her healthy kidney to Steve! This was as far as Steve or I would ever venture into any couples swapping arrangement, but it seemed so practical. Everybody could win!

Steve and I located the Triangle Parking Lot at the University of Washington and navigated our way through the imposing Medical

Center lobby. It reminded me of a bustling urban airport: shiny marble floors, interesting artwork, and people with more stories than we could imagine. There were faculty physicians strolling by in their crisp white lab coats, looking a bit imperious. There were the harried resident physicians and medical students in training, wearing blue scrub suits and rumpled lab coats, their pockets stuffed with reference handbooks, reflex hammers, and tongue blades. Then, there were dozens of "ordinary" people waiting in as many waiting areas; the range of humanity from the polished and clean to the raggedy flotsam and jetsam of Seattle: all comers, coming to Mecca for the gift of a miracle.

My stomach tightened as we walked past the clinic where I trained as a family practice resident. It was used as a specialty clinic now, but I had muscle memory and visceral memory of the University of Washington School of Medicine. It was as though my body and mind had an unconscious awareness of discomfort or personal risk, triggered by the memories of training as a medical professional in an intense environment. This wasn't uncommon. A friend of mine, an OB-Gyn physician, told me it had taken her almost a year before she could even drive in front of the Medical Center without experiencing a wave of nausea!

We found the Cafeteria Conference Room and were greeted by the pleasant young man who had helped me on the phone. He had originally scheduled Steve and me for two appointments: the Transplant Class required of all applicants and a second appointment on Valentine's Day, to meet with the transplant coordinator, social worker, and nephrologist. Due to a waiting period imposed by our health insurance company, the nice young man had phoned the week before to tell me that we couldn't schedule the comprehensive evaluation until April. I barely had the heart to tell Steve; he was counting so heavily on the transplant and wanted to do anything possible to hurry the process along. We were permitted to attend the class in spite of the insurance waiting period, and the gentleman promised us the first available April date for the more detailed appointment.

Steve and I signed in, collected pamphlets, and took our seats in the back of the room. There were about thirty people attending the meeting. Some were obviously patients; you could tell because they looked so ill. There were several patients with wheelchairs or other appliances, undoubtedly accommodations for diabetic neuropathy and related limb amputations. A show of hands confirmed that most of the patients were on dialysis. Others attending the class looked very healthy; I figured these were the partners or potential donors. But actually, one healthy-looking woman was there preparing for her *second* kidney transplant. One deaf patient "heard" the lecture through a sign language interpreter. Another man listened by way of a Spanish translator. This information was daunting enough as it was; imagine trusting an interpreter to make sure you got the information right!

The speaker informed us that she had been working in the transplant field for many years. There were numerous hoops to clear, she emphasized, and we were encouraged to jump through the hoops with impeccable care. The woman explained that a patient could receive a cadaver kidney from someone who had died but had designated themselves as an organ donor before death. This was often the case with auto accidents, where the communication occurred tacitly via the victim's driver's license. Or, a patient could receive a kidney from a living donor—usually a sibling, a friend, or a significant other. The speaker explained that a living donor kidney was preferable. After all, she told us, the living donor kidney hadn't been affected by some catastrophic process that "made it not living."

"Made it *not living*—for the love of God!" I whispered to Steve. "Everybody in this room understands *dead*. You can say *dead* here! We're all in this room because we either have End Stage Renal Disease, or we are intimately involved in the rugged life of someone who is practically dead already!"

The speaker went on to explain that all potential recipients were carefully screened to be certain they were medically suitable.

"We wouldn't want to give a kidney to someone with a very short life expectancy," she said. "You cannot smoke and receive a kidney transplant. And if you are very overweight, your surgical risk goes up. So you could be asked to lose weight before being considered to receive a transplant."

The morbidly obese young man sitting in front of us sank his teeth solidly into his French donut.

It occurred to me that Steve might not be considered "good enough" to receive a kidney. That decision would be made by people with the human foibles we all possess: jealousy, biases, transference. Would he be "worthy" in the eyes of the Transplant Team, or eliminated by some yet-undetermined health problem we didn't recognize? Steve and I exchanged a worried glance.

But the advantages of kidney transplant were summed up on one critical slide. For a diabetic patient on dialysis in Steve's age group, the average life expectancy was eight years. With a kidney transplant, however, that life expectancy increased to twenty years! Twenty years would see Brita through high school and college. Twenty years would get us onto that cruise ship. We could work with twenty years!

Steve and I moved to the cafeteria after the class for some cottage cheese and iced tea.

"What did you think?" I asked.

"I need a transplant," he answered with a determination in his eyes I'd never seen before.

"I get that," I said, "but you know that the new overnight dialysis shows a lot of promise, Steve. A transplant is a big surgery. Think of the cost of the anti-rejection drugs—$2000 per month—forever! And they didn't go into all the complications that are out there. If nocturnal dialysis works well, you might even choose *not* to have a transplant."

"I want a fucking kidney," Steve said with resolve. "I want *off the hose.*"

"I know," I sighed.

I wish the speaker could have sounded a bit more passionate, a little more connected with her audience. Maybe she could have thrown in some photographic slides of transplant recipients who had done well. Perhaps there could have been more of a welcome. Perhaps some minimal acknowledgement of the hell these patients had already endured, and the exhilarating potential of the new journey ahead. Perhaps she was just having a hectic day, but for us, this was *the* day that had been on our calendars for weeks. We hung on every word.

"So what do *you* think?" asked Steve.

"Oh, Steve," I replied, "I know you need a transplant, and we'll do anything we can to get you a new kidney."

My mind flashed back to the time when I was applying to the University of Washington Medical School. My mom had asked if it would help my application if she and my dad donated their bodies to the med school for research! The answer, of course, was no, but I wondered if anything might be done to "sweeten" Steve's candidacy in this situation.

"It's just that . . ." I sighed.

"It's just what?" pressed Steve.

"It's just that this is the university where I went to medical school—and where I did my residency training! I have some tough memories of this place."

Chapter Twenty

My experiences at the University of Washington came flooding back. I had decided to apply to medical school when my son Tim was only ten months old.

I remember the decision so clearly. I was sitting in my car at an intersection in the university district, thinking about a chance conversation I'd just had with a friend who had recently completed her first year of medical school. It sounded so exciting! The work I was doing as the Regional Family Planning Nurse Practitioner/Nurse Educator covering Washington, Oregon, Idaho, and Alaska—and serving as a nurse practitioner at Planned Parenthood—was wonderful. It was stimulating, meaningful work, and certainly the best possible job I could have had at age twenty-five. But where would I be at thirty-five?

Sitting in that intersection, I heard, not thought, but audibly *heard, "Well, you'll just have to go."*

I contacted the pre-med advisor the next day and charted my premed coursework: a year of biology, a year of physics, two years of premed chemistry, and some math. Interestingly, my nursing coursework would not count at all.

I began by taking two evening classes in calculus, one per quarter, and got a 4.0 in each class. The next step was chemistry, but there was no evening chemistry class offered. So I would run over to the university at mid-day for a chemistry class as a "lunch break," and then hurry back to work. By then, I was creeping out of my closet. Women with toddlers don't generally take calculus and chemistry on a recreational basis. My world was learning that I was a pre-med student.

The pre-med course work took three years to complete, given the responsibilities of my job and my family. Then, there was the MCAT—the grueling all-day Medical College Admissions Test covering biology, chemistry, physics, and scientific problem solving. I thought it was quite dreadful, until I learned that one of the other women in the room was in labor during the exam. At the time, the test was offered only twice a year; you didn't dare miss it!

Then, there was the application process: submitting letters of reference from sympathetic faculty and professional colleagues, and the in-person interview. I had practiced interview questions out loud in my car from the day I decided to apply to medical school: Why do you want to be a doctor? Why should we admit you, with all the stellar applicants we have? Why did you decide to become a nurse? Did you think you couldn't succeed as a physician? What is the most critical issue impacting healthcare today?

I made up the most difficult questions I could think of, and I practiced in the car until I nailed each answer. The interview was one thing over which I had at least partial control. My grades were fine; my MCAT scores were at least non-embarrassing. If I could just *get* to the interview, it was in my court! I bought the correct navy blue skirted suit to wear for the event.

Then, one snowy day in January of 1980, I received a phone call from the medical school office.

"Didn't you get our letter?" the woman asked. "We have you scheduled for an interview today!"

My heart plummeted. Of course I hadn't received the letter! It was snowing, and our suburban streets were icy. And Tim's father had just left in our pick-up truck with his cross-country skis in the back! I was home alone with three-year-old Tim, and no way to get to the interview—*my interview!*

"No, I did not receive your letter," I responded. "But please hold my spot. I will do everything humanly possible to get there today!"

I scrambled to get dressed. The tasteful navy suit was far too cold for that snowy day. I threw on a conservative turtleneck sweater, skirt, and a corduroy blazer. I hustled to get Tim dressed, praying that his dad would make it home in time for it to matter. By some stroke of fortune, Tim's dad did return and got me to the interview on time.

There were three panelists waiting for me: the admissions committee chairman, a current medical student, and a research professor on the medical school faculty. I plodded through the questions.

"What was the most important event in 1979," asked the chairman.

I discussed the hostage crisis in the Middle East.

"Did you become a nurse because you didn't think you could cut it as a physician?" another panelist asked.

"Not at all," I answered. "As a nurse practitioner, I learned that I love evaluating and treating patients. I appreciate the fact that I have real impact as a clinician. I can exercise a benevolent power in people's lives."

"You didn't think you were smart enough to succeed as a physician?"

"No," I replied. "I've pretty much been able to succeed at whatever I've set out to do."

Goodness! Was that me? Just the right amount of confidence, even arrogance! It worked. I learned in April of my acceptance to the University of Washington School of Medicine, with classes beginning in the fall of 1980.

The first two years of medical school were very tough for me: almost all science courses. The cadaver labs were intense, with four students around each dead body, four hours per session. The anatomy professor, who knew each of us by name before school even started, spoke in a heavy Transylvanian accent.

"Leenda," he would start, "if you were a little fairy standing on the peritoneum looking superiorly, what would you see in the region of the duodenum?"

Dr. Cornelius Rosse intimidated all of us. But we were to learn that he was one of the greats, and we loved him—in time.

I failed my first and only class in my entire academic career: biochemistry! I was embarrassed to my soul; I told only Andreas and Connie, my closest medical school friends. At the time, biochemistry hadn't been a formal prerequisite for med school, and I had never taken it. I learned quickly that three of my classmates had *PhDs* in biochemistry, solidly locking in *my* position at the bottom of the grading curve. I made up the deficiency with special tutoring from two marvelous professors, one a Nobel Laureate.

Andreas and I clung together for support, boosting each other with wit and irreverent humor. Neither of us would have made it without the other. Andreas would be asked a hypothetical patient-care question:

"What would you do in this clinical situation?" an instructor would ask.

"Get the patient to a real doctor!" Andreas would urge.

The two of us spent hours getting extra help in the Neuroanatomy Lab. Our professor would grab a Tupperware box containing a cadaver brain. Then, he'd slap the brain onto the lab counter and slice it open with a serrated bread knife.

"What is this structure?" the professor would ask.

"The lateral ventricle," we'd answer.

"And this?"

"The sella turcica."

Andreas would just look at me, roll his eyes, and say—in French, of course, "Where is the *nose*?"

So much detail was compressed into the first two years: anatomy, physiology, biochemistry, pharmacology. And most of my colleagues had hours more time to devote to studying: no kids, no part-time jobs (I worked for a small amount of money at the hospital, drawing patients' blood every morning before class).

The second two years were much better for me: all clinical rotations, working with patients in the various hospitals in Seattle in the full range of specialties: surgery, psychiatry, general medicine, obstetrics, and pediatrics, with additional rotations through the emergency room, and a host of electives.

I felt at home in the hospitals. At the very least, I was fluent in the language of medicine. I knew the abbreviations; I understood how patient care "flowed." I knew the hierarchy of personnel. I knew that I could contribute a therapeutic presence in a patient situation, and I wasn't afraid of asking questions.

What I didn't know—and what you simply can't know until experiencing it—was the reality of being on call. I'd arrive at the hospital at 5:30 a.m. on some mornings, and not leave the hospital until 5:30 p.m. the *next* afternoon! During that time, I'd "round" on patients, observe or help with surgeries, perform minor procedures, attend lectures, and write pages of patient chart notes. I'd see five different shifts of nurses during each on-call period. They'd all have been home to see their kids, to check their mail, to eat and sleep and go to the bathroom. Being on call was physically and mentally exhausting.

I learned that the quality of the hospital experience depended largely on which doctors and other students happened to be working with you. If your superior was an arrogant narcissist who wanted you to know for certain that your admission to medical school had been a terrible mistake, he—and that usually *was* a he—had the power to humiliate! An unkind remark could cut to the core, raising haunting doubts about our capabilities. We could, after all, kill someone! One day, Andreas said something wrong—he couldn't even remember what it was—and his attending physician took out a pair of scissors and *cut off Andreas' tie!*

But when it was good, and you were working with senior residents and attending physicians who loved medicine and loved to teach, it felt heady and joyful. We were all together on one team, and we had real power to use—on the side of good.

I remember one month, for example, being on an all-woman medical team. Our language was softer during that month. We didn't ask "Who are the players?" in referencing our patients. We didn't speak of aggressive medical interventions as a "full court press." We made evening rounds and "tucked our patients in" at night. I learned that there were many ways—many styles—in which to practice medicine.

I did my OB rotation at Madigan Army Hospital, a respectful culture of organized chaos where I delivered three babies on my first night and thirty little army babies over my month's rotation.

During my internal medicine rotation, I took care of the first AIDS patient admitted to a Seattle hospital. My presentation describing this gentleman's illness was included in Grand Rounds. It was attended by over a hundred physicians and students, all because they hungered for the new information. We were at the beginning of a new and fearsome era, and I was included in the team of helpers.

I loved medicine; I loved all fields of medicine. Not wanting to exclude whole areas or populations from my practice, I decided to pursue a residency in family medicine. I was accepted at my first choice of primary care programs: the University of Washington Family Medicine Residency Program.

Chapter Twenty-One

After a student graduates from the four years of medical school, he or she goes on to a residency program for more advanced training. The primary care programs are divided into three categories: internal medicine (treating adults only), pediatrics (treating patients from infants through adolescents), and family medicine (treating individuals from birth to death, including obstetrics).

Or a student goes into general surgery, orthopedic surgery, anesthesia, obstetrics and gynecology, or psychiatry. Medical subspecialties such as gastroenterology, endocrinology, or nephrology, usually follow internal medicine residencies. There are surgical sub-specialties as well, also requiring further years of training after a general surgery foundation. The different programs have their own requirements for periodic board certification. All programs require a minimum of three years beyond the four years of medical school, and everyone is required to earn continuing medical education credits for the duration of their career. After all, medical education is a career-long endeavor.

Primary care doctors are the "first line" doctors who evaluate patients, treat most conditions, and refer the most complicated cases to the appropriate specialists. The University of Washington is nationally reputed for its excellence in primary care education, and primary care residencies are highly competitive.

That said, however, there is an arrogance conveyed by certain specialists—a sense of superiority over the first-line doctors in the trenches. When I was weighing my residency choices, one OB-Gyn specialist advised me, "If you go into family medicine, you'll learn how to do a lot of things—*poorly*."

It is true that primary care requires far more *breadth,* and specialties require far more *depth* of knowledge. Primary care doctors must be good "scanners," analyzing the big picture, reading between the lines for their patients' unspoken subtexts, and culling out what is clinically most urgent for the patient. Sometimes the primary care provider serves as a "broker," finding the best specialist for a particular patient. It's challenging work. Most headaches aren't brain tumors and most skin spots aren't malignant melanomas—but they can be! Knowing when to worry requires considerable skill and information. But it can be hard to cut through the biases of other physicians, especially as a resident physician at Mecca.

Once during a surgical rotation, I was assisting with a breast cancer operation. The surgeon was "pimping" me—the term we used for asking absurdly detailed questions, probably to pass the time, possibly for his own entertainment. He asked me about a specific morsel of trivia, and I said I didn't know the answer.

"A *surgical* resident would know the answer to that question, Dr. Gromko," he said.

"Well," I replied, "I'm not a surgical resident, Sir. I'm part of your *referral* base."

The Operating Room fell silent: one point for me!

I believe there will always be a need for excellent generalists. I know without a doubt that I could not do the work of some of Steve's specialist physicians. But could *they* move through *my* day in family medicine: diabetes to sinusitis, to vaginal bleeding, to anxiety in a nine-year-old, to a diaphragm fitting, to depression, to a geriatric patient with mini-strokes, to a skin biopsy of an abnormal mole, to a migraine, to a woman's health care exam, to morbid obesity, to the drainage of a skin abscess, to alcoholism in a bipolar transgendered patient? Probably not.

Residency was even more difficult than medical school. We rotated nearly every month to a new service, covering the gambit of medical and surgical areas, plus inpatient psychiatry, OB, the Emergency Room, and a raft of electives. In addition, we saw our own "continuity" patients in the Family Medicine Clinic: patients who called us "Doctor" from day one, and expected that we'd know what to do from the very beginning.

Residency, of course, required being on call. "Call" was even more burdensome than as a medical student. In medical school, we might be responsible for admitting one or two patients a night. "Admitting" a patient meant taking the patient's history, performing a physical examination, formulating a treatment plan, writing orders for procedures and medical tests, and writing exhaustive chart notes. In residency, we might admit as many as *ten* patients, often working through the entire night. We learned that three hours of sleep is far better than no sleep at all. I learned that "a shower is worth an hour" of sleep. But it was simply exhausting.

So often, I felt that patients deserved more than I had the capacity to give them. I remember one afternoon, having just completed my thirty-fifth hour on duty with no sleep whatsoever. I had just lost a patient: a terribly complicated sixty-year-old man who died in the Surgical Intensive Care Unit because of a ruptured colon. He died in spite of maximal surgical support and the maximal capacity of the ventilator (breathing machine). His eighty-five-year-old mother came to visit him, and to learn from me that her son had just expired. I felt it was appropriate that I was the one to tell her. I had spoken with her many times before, and I had been intimately involved in her son's care. It's just that when you are eight-five, and you lose your only child, I think you should have the benefit of someone with more fortitude than a weary intern on hour thirty-five! I comforted the grieving mother the best I could, and guided her into the loving arms of one of the nuns on duty.

Occasionally, we truly had more responsibility than we were competent to handle. One night as an intern (first-year resident), I remember being the only physician on shift at the University of Washington ER. My supervising physician was sleeping at home. A moderately ill-appearing woman came in for evaluation. By some divine intervention, I drew a blood culture; if she had an infection in her bloodstream, the culture would show this in a day or two. Her other lab tests, all available on a stat basis, were normal. I telephoned my supervising physician, awakening him at five a.m. We discussed her case, and he said to send the patient home. I did so, with instructions that she should return immediately if anything worsened. Later in the day when her blood culture grew out meningococcus, a particularly deadly bacterium, the ER staff contacted her immediately and brought her back to the hospital for "big gun" antibiotics. I honestly believe that woman would have died without that fortuitous blood culture.

It seemed as though we as resident physicians "couldn't tie our shoes right" during the day, but became stellar clinicians at night—when the private physicians were home in bed.

One night in the Coronary Care Unit, I admitted a cardiac patient displaying a potpourri of heart rhythms. She had come to the hospital with an astonishingly high blood level of the heart medicine digoxin. I phoned her cardiologist at two a.m. After all, I had never seen a digoxin level of *nine* (normal might be a level of one ng/ml), and I really didn't know what to do for the patient. I worried that her heart rhythms would degenerate into more ominous patterns, like potentially lethal ventricular fibrillation or asystole.

But the cardiologist was angry.

"*You* manage it!" he challenged. "I don't want to be bothered with this kind of shit at two in the morning!"

He slammed down the phone.

"Wow," I thought, "*this* kind of shit? This is good shit!"

In retrospect, I wonder if the cardiologist even knew what to do. Sometimes, anger and arrogance are foils for ignorance. He was probably as scared as I was.

Truly, in most situations, patients did get good care. Our attending physicians were generally top-notch. As in anything in life, the bad days can stick indelibly in your memory. It is also fair to point out that residency programs have been modified over the last twenty years, to limit the number of sleepless hours and to restrict the number of patients admitted by a resident in any given call night. And today, I would never have been alone as an intern, as the single physician in the University Hospital Emergency Room.

Chapter Twenty-Two

If my residency had been "simply" a barrage of detail, difficult work, and physical and mental exhaustion, I probably would have managed through it pretty well. I was effective as a clinician, familiar with the hospital culture, and I really enjoyed helping people through their crises.

But my residency experience took a serious turn for the worse about midway through the second year, and morphed into what a colleague called the "Story of Job Residency." A litany of horrors descended on my family and me—not because of the residency, but always within its context.

In November 1985, while rotating through the Veterans Administration Hospital as a second-year resident on the internal medicine service, I was "found down" on my call room floor. I remember having had a particularly busy day, with many patients admitted through the night. I remember going to bed for a nap before it would be time for our team's early morning blood draw. I recall getting up and going out of my call room to get some cold water at the drinking fountain just outside. My next recollection was seeing a startled Asian cleaning man standing over me. He had discovered me—out cold—on my call room floor. I remember only fragments of the next few hours: my senior resident drawing my blood and giving me juice to drink, other residents commenting on the red marks they found on my neck and arms.

Had I been assaulted? There was no evidence of this, but I truly did not know what had happened. The time—about an hour and a half—had been completely edited from my memory.

I was transferred by ambulance to the University of Washington Hospital where I was admitted with the presumptive diagnosis of seizure. I had never had a seizure before. A new seizure at age thirty-five carried the possibility of a brain tumor!

But my head CT was normal, as were my EKG and EEG (brain wave test). One cardiologist postulated that I might have had an electrical misstep in my heart rhythm. But a seizure, while not witnessed, was felt to be the most likely diagnosis. (I was to learn that anyone can have a seizure, given the "right" conditions. In my case, it might have been a "brain misfire" at the interface of wakefulness and sleep.) I was discharged home on Dilantin, a common anticonvulsant. I was also advised not to drive for the next six months, a factor which would require me to rearrange some of my clinical rotations.

Several days after starting the Dilantin, I developed a high fever and a lobster-red rash that covered my body from head to toe. Vomiting and dangerously dehydrated, I was again admitted to University Hospital, this time for a severe allergic reaction to Dilantin. I was switched to Phenobarbital, which had the capacity to prevent seizures but was markedly sedating. I would have to take a month off from the residency program to recover, which played havoc with the other residents' schedules as well as my own.

While I was in the hospital being treated for the allergic reaction, my seventy-one-year-old father, normally a healthy and robust insurance salesman, was also admitted to University Hospital. Never a complainer, he was brought in by ambulance with acute abdominal pain. A gallstone had become lodged in the duct leading from his pancreas into the duodenum, creating an aggressive inflammation: pancreatitis. The pancreas, an organ located in the upper mid abdomen, has a variety of functions; producing insulin and glucagon to control blood sugar, and producing a number of enzymes that aid in the digestion of proteins and fats. With an obstruction in the duct leading out of the pancreas, the organ begins to digest itself!

My father became perilously ill, requiring a ventilator within a couple of days. He would be trapped on that ventilator for a full three months, first with a tube going down his throat, and later with a tracheostomy tube surgically implanted in his neck. He developed a "pseudocyst," a mass in his belly the size of a volleyball that would later be surgically removed. He developed sepsis: a life-threatening infection in his bloodstream.

At his admission to the hospital, my father exhibited nine of the eleven "Ranson's Criteria" which defined the severity of pancreatitis. His case was presented before surgical Grand Rounds in front of over one hundred physicians and students. It seemed that nobody thought he would live.

I believe our family handled my dad's horrible illness with as much dignity as a family could muster. My mom, who didn't drive, would take two buses to the University Hospital, arriving each morning at nine and leaving at three in the afternoon. I would come earlier in the morning, also by bus because of the seizure-imposed driving restrictions, and spend some time with my father in the ICU before my own clinic began. Then, I'd spend an hour or two with him in the evening before my husband would pick me up at nine p.m. We would bring Tim in on the weekends, sometimes wearing his hockey gear. My sister and her family would spend time with Dad as well.

During my dad's admission, I learned that creating a family presence—showing that we as a family were present and involved—translated into better care. We played soothing, lyrical music on a portable tape recorder. When possible, we would turn the fluorescent lights down low. The respiratory therapists would tell us how much they appreciated coming into my dad's room. The music provided calming relaxation, and our presence conveyed to everyone that *this* patient was a respected part of a family, a person who *mattered*.

But even this didn't always work. Because the residents rotated every month and my dad was in the hospital for a full five months, we experienced the loving compassion of most resident teams—and the dangerous indifference of another.

One day, I stood washing dishes at my kitchen sink when the hospital called. My dad was suddenly much worse. I rushed to the hospital to see my father spouting blood from a giant blowhole in his neck. His tracheostomy tube had become dislodged; my dad was agitated, pulling at his neck. He was flanked by a surgical resident and a family practice resident from my program.

"Stop that!" the surgical resident admonished my dad. "If you don't settle down, we'll have to *paralyze* you!"

I knew what the surgeon meant; they'd give my dad a short-acting sedative or muscle relaxant, or maybe a medication which would paralyze his muscles *temporarily.* But I'm positive that my dad thought they would paralyze his whole body forever—and I was furious!

"Don't you *ever* talk to my father that way! That is no way to speak to him—or any other patient!"

I motioned the surgeon to a side room.

"He can't possibly understand what you mean. It's inappropriate, and it's cruel!"

"You shouldn't be in here," responded the surgeon. "We can't have family in here."

The family practice resident whispered to the surgeon that I was a physician too. I stood my ground and didn't move; the surgeon walked out, with others attending to my dad.

On another occasion, I watched as my father developed the classic signs and symptoms of pneumonia: rapid, labored breathing; cough; high fever; decreased mental lucidity. I phoned the surgical resident personally, but antibiotics were not started until the next evening—a full twenty-four hours later.

When I asked why the delay, the surgical resident offered, "Oh, it won't matter."

"Well, you don't wait to cut on an acute abdomen!" I countered.

I tempered my response and said no more. This doctor was stupid and indifferent. I believe that *if you're going to be arrogant, you'd better be right!* But I didn't want to antagonize this doctor and compromise my father's care.

I was reminded of the very real medical vulnerability patients can experience. As an advocate for my father, I was seen as a family member, not as a physician colleague. There was a difference in power. The overworked, exhausted residents at University Hospital could advocate for my father, and certainly, most did. Or, they could ignore him or even abuse him.

In the midst of all this hell, I was still functioning as a resident physician myself, with my own clinic patients and hospital rotations. Our family felt so public, so exposed. One of my faculty members made a comment that I was spending too much time with my father.

"I'm not aware that it is interfering with my work," I said. "Besides, he's my *father.*"

The instructor replied, "But that's just the point, Linda. He's your father—not your *son!*"

What impropriety was being implied here? The people who were grading me were also judging me. I didn't expect them to be supportive necessarily; I just never expected them to *aim!* It was a personally vulnerable time.

My life was unbalanced; my dad in the ICU, my mom barely coping. My own health was in question, and though there were no new seizure events, I experienced the overwhelming, mind-dulling sedation of the Phenobarbital. Money was frightfully tight; my marriage began to unravel.

Riding on the bus to the University of Washington one morning I thought of a powerful advocate: Margy Anderson, my dear counselor in medical school who had run the support group for former nurses which Connie and I had attended. Margy had died of metastatic breast cancer years earlier.

"Margy," I thought, sitting very still with my eyes closed. "Margy, what on earth should I do now?"

Audibly—again, audibly, not simply a thought, I heard: "Do the best you can and love will back you up."

My eyes startled open: *Do the best you can, and love will back you up.* What a profound message! I recognized that my best was not inconsequential. I knew I carried a moral obligation to do my best work. After all, I was given this tremendous opportunity to become a physician—to do the work I loved. And the concept of "backup" is significant in medicine. Your backup physician might be an attending physician or a senior resident who knew more than you did. In any case, *my* backup was "love." I was humbled, comforted, and confused all at once.

But even after that providential message, my life continued to bring challenge after challenge. I felt as though I was standing in front of a pitching machine! Over the next few months, I came down with shingles, requiring IV antiviral medications. Then, I experienced a near-fatal asthma attack that took me to the ICU via Medic One. The skilled paramedic who literally saved my life told me that he had considered performing a crichothyroidotomy—putting a needle *through* the front of my neck—in my bedroom! I stayed in the ICU overnight and in the hospital for several more days. My asthma required industrial doses of the steroid, prednisone. Some nights when back at work, I would write my patient chart notes hooked up to a nebulizer for a breathing treatment in the preemie center or the ICU. My asthma had been exacerbated by a "pansinusitis," a severe sinus infection. The surgery to correct this was done by way of local anesthesia and sedation. I was fully awake during the operation, holding absolutely still as I listened to the crunch of surgical instruments inside my head and face.

As my marriage deteriorated, my husband and I decided to file for divorce. We sold our home; sadly, the only home Tim knew, and moved to separate apartments, sharing Tim's care. By the time my residency ended, I was waiting for the locusts to appear!

But, blessedly, the residency did end.

My father went home after five long months at University Hospital. He went on to live five more "bonus years" before dying of a massive stroke. To this day, he was the sickest person I have *ever* seen in my career—that is to say, the sickest person who actually recovered.

So, in discussing kidney transplant surgery at the University of Washington, I explained to Steve that the university bore some rough associations for me. Medical school and residency were difficult enough without the litany of personal challenges I confronted. And it was impossible for me to compartmentalize the family and health issues, to separate them out from the medical school and residency experiences. They were inextricably intertwined, messy memories.

The Transplant Class brought the experiences colliding back. Could I return to the scene of such composite personal suffering?

Yes, I concluded. I would do the best I could, as I had done before, and trust in the power of love to back me up.

Chapter Twenty-Three

At the end of January 2008, Steve had had the second of two operations to create a dialysis fistula in his forearm. The fistula would grow into a giant blood vessel, and could be used for dialysis in place of the riskier central line catheter in his internal jugular vein.

After the surgery, Steve's hands became "twitchy" again, and he felt vaguely "off." I feared the worst. Then, he had a fall in the bedroom—no injury sustained, but a fall nonetheless.

While Steve had experienced years of *high* blood pressure, we were suddenly having difficulty keeping his blood pressure high *enough.* One day, as Steve's blood pressure hovered around 80/50, I tried giving him oral fluids to raise his blood pressure. Then, I tried repositioning his body with his legs elevated—supported on my shoulders to move fluid from his extremities into his core circulation. I finally gave him saline through his central line—not your typical family first aid. But we were on Bainbridge Island, and I didn't want Steve passing out.

I realized on that day that Steve was too fragile to move his dialysis treatments to my office, as we had negotiated. But my other concern was that we were treating a number of patients with MRSA in my office: patients with skin abscesses due to antibiotic-resistant staphylococcal infections. I would never forgive myself if Steve developed a MRSA-related central line infection while dialyzing in my office.

Was I selling out, acquiescing to Steve? Perhaps so; I had every right to insist that Steve compromise. But at the moment, at least, I was the stronger of the two of us, the one able to make the sacrifice. I returned the dialysis chair to the Kidney Center, the chair that Neves had been so kind to deliver.

Life moved ahead: Brita went snowboarding for a week in Jackson Hole, Steve traveled to Minnesota for a two-day business trip in February, and I sold my Belltown condo. I signed us all up for a family membership at Island Fitness; Steve could at least walk on a treadmill and I could take spinning classes. In spite of dialysis—and because of it—we were making our way as a new family.

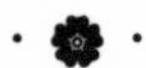

In March 2008, Steve was slated to attend IHRSA, the International Health Club and Racquet Sports Association Conference and Trade Show, to be held in San Diego. IHRSA presented a varied mix of the fitness industry: plenty of spandex and lycra, perky aerobic goddesses, and broad-shouldered muscle men oozing testosterone. You could find anything associated with the operation of health clubs: protein bars, gym bags, balance balls, towel supplies, stretching bands, and antiseptic wash to prevent the spread of bacteria.

But the real thrust of the show was Steve's interest: fitness equipment like treadmills, stair climbers, upper-body cranking machines, and the full range of strength-training equipment. Steve, now under a product contract with the Cybex Corporation, was actually an industry titan with decades of experience and the personal contacts to prove it. Curious, really: this still-rounded, anemic, balding man on a kidney machine was a veritable fitness icon!

Because attending IHRSA was an industry requirement for Steve, I would go with him to the conference at the San Diego Marriott as his dialysis assistant. We'd "simply" perform the dialysis treatments in our hotel room at night. Since Steve was to be out of town for four days, skipping treatments was not considered; four days without treatment could be a life-and-death matter.

We loaded the kidney machine, weighing exactly one hundred pounds in its aluminum travel box. Plus another eighty pounds of gear—IV tubing, kidney machine cartridges, syringes, Heparin, dressing materials—all in a duffel bag. Steve mainly directed this operation; I was the Sherpa, grateful that my years of strength training were paying off. We proceeded to the Alaska Airlines counter with our American Disabilities Act literature in hand. As the medical equipment was required to sustain Steve's life, we could not be charged extra for its priority travel.

Arriving at the Marriott, we were relieved to learn that the other critical portion of our supplies, the eight boxes of dialysate bags, had been delivered by NxStage.

On our first day in San Diego, Steve saw dozens of friends. He was obviously well known and well liked, with a line-up of individuals seeking his time and opinions. I imagine that the news of Steve's kidney failure spread rapidly through the fitness community; many were amazed to see Steve there at all.

We met one of Steve's oldest friends, Don Gronachan, for dinner. "The Gronk," as Steve had christened him years before, was an exercise physiologist with PhD-caliber training. He ran a division in a multi-million-dollar company manufacturing high-level physical therapy equipment.

Steve and Don reminisced after dinner about their early days when they had worked together at Cybex. Don—all of five-feet-two-inches—was to present a clinical lecture to the Cybex sales force, and Steve was to introduce him. Steve felt the salespeople might be bored unless Don did something memorable to engage them.

Drawing from Don's impressive gymnastics background, Steve coached, "Hey, do a few back flips on the way to the podium!"

Don looked incredulous. "You're kidding, right?"

"No, really,' Steve directed, "Just do it!"

In his business suit and tie, The Gronk executed a flawless series of back flips, and a round-off—ending with a Mary Lou Retton finish immediately in front of the podium. The crowd went wild!

Don's credibility with the sales force was cemented. Steve had a knack for setting up unorthodox fun, and somehow, people trusted his guidance. Again and again, I would hear stories about how Steve's knowledge and instincts had made a difference in people's careers.

Predictably, Don was fascinated by the technology of Steve's dialysis. "Come on along," we urged. "Join us for Steve's treatment! It'll be fun, as long as you don't mind watching Steve's blood running in and out of his body."

The three of us finished our dinner and took the elevator to our sixteenth-floor room overlooking the bay. Steve and I explained the basics of the kidney machine to Don, and I set out to triple-check our supplies.

"Oh, no," I sighed. "There's one thing I forgot. I hope there's nothing else."

"What?" asked Steve, with obvious concern.

"Well, you know the tubing that carries the waste to the sink in our bathroom at home? It's not long enough for *this* room, and I don't have any extension tubing."

I glanced around the room, and found a watertight wastebasket. It would probably hold about a gallon. I called room service and ordered another. Then, we placed the two containers on the veranda, in case of a dribble, and taped the waste hose to one of the receptacles.

"We could just run the waste line off the balcony," Steve offered.

"Oh, no we won't," I replied. "This is the Marriott, you buffalo!"

And Don added, "It wouldn't be the *first* time Steve Williams peed off the balcony of a Marriott hotel!"

Oh my. We proceeded with the dialysis treatment, as Steve and Don talked into the evening. I'd jump up now and again to empty another wastebasket of dialysis fluid and "urine" into the bathtub—a total of about thirty liters in all, in a low-tech bucket brigade.

The trade show started in earnest the next morning. All the industry leaders were there. We found Roy Simonson, Steve's business partner, who had designed dozens of pieces of exercise and strength training equipment, yet exercised his own extremely fit body by dragging a steel chain over his shoulder as he'd run up a mountainside with his wife Cindy. Cindy was a legend herself, once skiing down the face of a Jackson Hole run and giving birth to their first child only minutes later! The Italian executives from Technogym had arrived from Cezena in their impeccably tailored business suits. Their enormous exhibit sprawled around a central espresso café serving cappuccino and biscotti; their company's new products included a line of stretching equipment so elegant that the pieces could have passed for fine furniture.

Cybex, Precor, LifeFitness, and Startrack all came to the show to display their newest wares, and to give participants a chance to try the equipment in person. There were spinning classes and Pilates classes. A circle of participants tried the new upper body Krank machine, as instructors urged them to "Keep on krankin!"

I took a couple of classes, walked the trade show floor, and met plenty of Steve's friends—folks he had known for decades. It was great to see Steve in his element, where he was recognized as a well-known and well-respected contributor.

Later, I ventured out to shop and explore sunlit San Diego. The next morning, I collapsed like a rag doll in the elegance of the Tiki Spa, soaking up a rare opportunity to be rubbed and buttered—far away from the demands of business, medicine, and family.

We had another dinner out, this time at the Fish Market, with a dozen industry leaders. Jim Croft and Dan Ashcraft were guests who straddled both of Steve's industries: audio and fitness. Jim is an inventor in the loudspeaker industry and Dan owns a leading industrial design firm. Steve described both of these men as geniuses in their respective, overlapping fields.

I had met Jim and Dan two-and-a-half years earlier, when Steve had hosted a wedding reception for Jim and his new bride Pamela at Steve's Bainbridge Island home. What an event *that* was: significant in the fact that I even stayed with Steve through it!

Steve is an excellent cook, but he hadn't planned for enough supplies. Only six months into our relationship, there I was, serving as Steve's scullery maid. I was desperately trying to turn our loaves and fishes into enough food—with abundant coaching from Steve and Brita on "how we do it."

At one point in the party, I heard there was a problem outside on the front lawn. It turned out that the automatic lawn sprinklers had activated, showering water into a guest's open Ferrari convertible! Thinking it was a medical problem, i.e., something *important,* I bolted through what I thought was an open patio door. Instead, it was a large picture window. I hit that window hard, knocking off my glasses and dropping to my knees. I was a bit disoriented at the shock of the impact. Of course I felt completely ridiculous! Here we were hosting a party for all of these wonderful, important friends of Steve, and I was thunking into a picture window like a misguided robin! The graciousness of Dan and Jim helped me feel at least a bit less stupid: Dan even suggested we etch my name—and those of any other victims—on the window pane.

Steve's friends at IHRSA were all extraordinary people: gifted in their fields, witty and creative, and invested in their friendships with Steve. I was being welcomed as an honored participant, the valued wife of a deeply regarded friend.

Steve and I had one more dialysis run on the night before we left San Diego. This time, we just sat on the big bed and watched TV. We ordered a room-service dinner of comfort foods; disavowing all guilt about the pint of Haagen-Daaz butter pecan ice cream we devoured.

It had been a significant trip for us. Steve and I demonstrated to each other that we could manage dialysis on the road. Steve was able to conduct his work without a major intrusion from Kidney World. We felt victorious, reclaiming yet another piece of our lives that End Stage Renal Disease might well have taken.

Chapter Twenty-Four

By mid-March 2008, Steve's fistula had finally matured enough to begin using it for dialysis. After two surgeries to create the fistula, i.e., connecting a forearm artery to a forearm vein, the vein had grown impressively. This had tremendous meaning. For one thing, dialysis done through a fistula is more effective in removing the body's poisons. A fistula is also less likely to become infected than a central line like the one Steve had in his jugular vein. We felt fortunate that Steve's central line had functioned perfectly, and without infection, for an eventual total of eight months.

It would be healthier for Steve to have the central line removed, and it would simplify his life as well. No more showers with quart-sized freezer bags duct-taped over the central line ports! (Steve announced that he would be able to wash his right armpit!) Plus, the red and blue plastic ports hanging from Steve's jugular vein had become a rather hideous reminder of Steve's compromised health. If feeling badly much of the time wasn't enough, Steve had only to glance at the ports dangling unnaturally from his upper chest to remind himself of his End Stage Renal Disease.

Just as we had trained to do home dialysis through the central line at the Kidney Center in Seattle, we had to train to use the fistula at the

Kidney Center as well. After all the work that had been done to create it, the fistula had to be carefully guarded. Dialysis via fistula requires inserting two giant needles into the fistula and hooking them to the kidney machine by way of IV tubing. As with the two central line ports, one needle led blood away from Steve's body and into the machine; the other returned the blood after it was filtered.

For perspective, Steve would give himself insulin using delicate 31-gauge needles (the larger the gauge, the smaller the needle). We might administer antibiotics in my office through larger 21-gauge needles. The fistula needles, on the other hand, looked like pipes: 15-gauge needles so large that you could see their central core throughout! They were more like trochars or spears than needles, with menacingly sharp tips. I had had plenty of practice in drawing blood, giving injections, and starting IVs, but I had never plunged a 15-gauge pipe into anyone's arm! Let alone, into my husband's arm with the precious fistula to be protected at all cost.

We learned the concept of "buttonholing." If you slide the needle into the fistula in exactly the same angle and direction each time, you ultimately create a tunnel for its insertion. Running along the same little pathway, the needles will ultimately become relatively easy to insert, with less risk of perforation (piercing the back wall of the vein and creating a leak). The "buttonhole" is similar in concept to the hole in a pierced ear; it heals in such a way that a blunt earring tip can move through the hole without requiring sharp penetration. Ultimately, one can move from sharp fistula needles to blunt buttonhole needles. Personally, I felt "blunt" was a misnomer; the blunt needles looked quite threatening as well.

My early attempts at inserting fistula needles into Steve's arm were encouraging. Then, I hit a snag; I couldn't get the needles in to save my soul. This was infuriating because a fistula is so large you can *see* it protruding through the skin surface. Sometimes, I could get the needle into the vein but the blood would clot off, unusable. Occasionally, I would just miss altogether. Other times, I could get one needle in, but not the other. We both recognized that we couldn't take Steve's blood out of his body without returning it. The process was physically painful for Steve, in spite of the local anesthetics we used. It was tough on my ego as well.

The stress began to mount again: the 6:20 a.m. ferries, the challenges of training, the bludgeoning commute, dialysis on top of my medical practice, dialysis on top of Steve's work, plus all of life's normal responsibilities like Brita and even my mom. We felt we were doing nothing particularly well, just barely managing. Brita and I would have verbal arguments, which we handled reasonably well. Steve, on the other hand, hated these conflicts—calling them "shitstorms." He bitterly hated the fact that his kidney disease impacted all of us. But there was no denying it: Steve's kidney disease *did* impact all of us. It's just that it wasn't his fault.

Our tender new marriage was strained. I bought Dr. John Gottman's book, *The Seven Principles for Making Marriage Work.* Gottman claimed that you could predict which couples were doomed to divorce early in their marriages, simply by observing their interactions. He cautioned about what he termed "The Four Horsemen of the Apocalypse." The four horsemen of marital discord were: criticism, contempt, defensiveness, and stonewalling—all signs of trouble to come. As Steve and I poured through Gottman's book, we felt those horsemen circling. We'd quiz each other of the names of the four horsemen, but we'd invariably launch into the names of the Teletubbies instead!

I guess if your horsemen are Po, Dipsy, LaLa, and TinkyWinky, there could be hope. But it seemed far too early to tell.

Chapter Twenty-Five

On April 9, 2008, Steve and I went to the University of Washington for our initial appointment with the transplant team. We met with the nurse coordinator, the nutritionist, the social worker, and the nephrologist. The nurse coordinator explained that she had worked with the program for almost thirty years. She and the social worker emphasized the shortage of cadaver donors, the need to be constantly available in case one found a match, and the rugged medical regimen which followed a transplant. They discussed the deluge of costly medications, and the necessity for frequent early-morning appointments. I imagine you *have* to be regimented if your work is transplanting vital organs, and the team delivered a businesslike, almost dispassionate approach.

I had learned earlier that my type B blood type would not be compatible with Steve's type A blood, and therefore I could not be his kidney donor. Steve would require a donor of blood group A or O. We asked about the couples match, where two or more couples share in the process of swapping compatible organs. The team represented that the University of Washington program was not yet set up to facilitate couples matching, but it was theoretically possible and had been done at other centers.

It was clear that it was preferable to "bring your own kidney" in the form a living kidney donor, like a sympathetic family member or friend. Steve had a couple of friends who had volunteered, but it was all too early in the process to know. Factors like compatibility and sincerity can be elusive. And it is a *kidney*, after all!

I thought of Steve's blunt comment to Dr. Thakur: "Who do I have to blow to get a kidney?"

Thankfully, Steve presented a more formal approach at the University of Washington. But it put a different spin on our lives. When compassionate people would ask, "Is there anything I can do to help?" we were ready to ask them their blood type and offer up a Living Donor brochure.

We learned that the average wait for a cadaver donor compatible with Steve's blood type was two years. While two years doesn't sound like such a long time, *we* considered that two out of five in-center dialysis patients *die* within a span of two years. You could theoretically get a match, but not live to receive it. We expected that Steve's chances of survival were considerably greater on home dialysis, for a host of reasons. But clearly, time was of the essence.

The transplant team informed us that Steve would be considered as a transplant candidate, but he had to be medically cleared and financially approved first. The nephrologist then performed a physical exam, after which Steve received an update of his immunizations and a TB test. We ended the day with a trip to the lab for the collection of *nineteen* vials of Steve's blood.

The most critical question looming ahead of Steve's medical clearance for a kidney transplant was this: would the University of Washington cardiologists require another cardiac catheterization (angiogram) to assess the blood vessels supplying Steve's heart? The angiogram carried risks of its own—risks of stroke, heart rhythm disturbances, even death—so the question was not trivial.

Like most diabetic kidney patients, Steve was no stranger to heart disease. Eight years earlier at age fifty, Steve had seen his primary care internist, Dr. Tauben, for a comprehensive physical examination. Steve, while heavy, had always been quite fit—a formidable racquetball player and always a gym rat. But he had become uncharacteristically winded on a day hike, and was haunted by his father's death of congestive heart failure at only fifty-six. Dr. Tauben sent Steve to consult with Dr. Ali, a cardiologist.

In her soft-spoken but business-like manner, Dr. Ali announced that Steve's EKG was abnormal. She moved directly to perform an urgent cardiac catheterization. The cardiac "cath" is an invasive X-ray study during which the cardiologist inserts a large catheter into the femoral artery in the groin and feeds the catheter up into the heart itself. By injecting dye through the catheter, the cardiologist is able to outline each blood vessel supplying the heart. Most importantly, the study demonstrates any narrowing of blood vessels: stenoses where blockages may have occurred, or will likely occur in the future.

Dr. Ali discovered significant narrowing in two vessels: Steve's left anterior descending artery (LAD) and his right coronary artery (RCA). The LAD supplies the big left ventricle, the chamber which is *the* most critical in pumping blood to the rest of the body. The LAD is so important in cardiac function that it is often dubbed the "widow maker"; a sudden blockage of the LAD can virtually disable the heart and result in sudden death.

In spite of an 80–90 percent narrowing of both the LAD and the RCA (which supplies the lower part of the heart), Steve's heart muscle function had been well maintained. He had not had a heart attack or heart muscle damage—yet.

Steve's cardiac cath illustrated an excellent argument for exercise. It is thought that with an active lifestyle, a person can build extra blood vessels to serve the heart muscle. These "collateral" vessels are thought to act as a safety net, providing alternative pathways through which the heart muscle is nourished.

The other significant lesson of Steve's angiogram is the effect of diabetes on the heart. Diabetics are clearly at higher risk for heart disease than are their non-diabetic counterparts. Additionally, the symptoms of heart disease are often less obvious in the diabetic. Newer guidelines for cholesterol management recommend that the diabetic patient be considered to have the *same,* i.e., higher, cardiac risk as someone who has *already* had a heart attack, even if there is no known heart disease.

Steve underwent heart surgery on September 3, 1999, a few days after his cardiac catheterization. The surgery was a two-vessel coronary artery bypass graft, or CABG. During a bypass, veins of the leg or chest are "harvested" to create a bridge around a narrowed portion of the coronary artery, thus increasing the blood flow to the area.

Steve recalls being in the hospital for only two nights after his CABG. He was in a ward with "three other poor schmucks who had also just had their chests cracked": three other previously robust, middle-aged men who clutched their red heart-shaped pillows as they attempted to grasp their own new realities.

Steve, impressed by his "come to Jesus" CABG, remembers trying to be the model patient, walking a quarter mile on his first day home on Bainbridge Island. Steve was assisted in the first post-operative week by his earliest childhood friend, Larry Running, another of Steve's friends who seemed willing to drop their own lives for a while to come and help out.

Things went smoothly for the first few days, but then Steve began to feel vaguely worse. His appetite was lagging, and he couldn't have a bowel movement—not an uncommon problem after surgery, where narcotics used to control pain can also slow the bowel motility.

He telephoned his surgeon's office and was advised to go to the emergency room of the nearest hospital, not the Seattle hospital where the surgery had been performed. Steve said he was treated in the ER "like a post-op whiner." But there had been no blood work, no X-rays, and no prescriptions offered. He was simply released home again presumably to continue his whining.

During the early post-operative period, Brita was lovingly housed by old friends George and Cheryl Mead. George was the son of my junior high school math teacher. George and Cheryl had spent countless hours with Steve when they all rented homes in the Hamptons, but their connection went clear back to high school. George and Cheryl were designated to be the couple who would raise Brita if Steve hadn't made it through the surgery.

In the second post-operative week, Steve was assisted by another old friend, Terry Donofrio. During that week, things turned critically worse. Steve felt terrible; he became bloated and couldn't walk well. His chest began to hurt much more, and he still couldn't move his bowels.

Terry drove Steve to the nearby ER a second time. This time Steve was sent for a chest X-ray, and the experience was harrowing.

"The X-ray technician put his arms under my armpits and pulled me off the gurney and onto the X-ray table. I heard a loud crack, and felt my sternum (breast bone) 'give.' And after that time, my sternum moved as though it was made of two separate parts—with the right side and the left side of the bone moving independently."

"Was that painful?" I asked.

"Oh, *terribly* painful," Steve answered. "But Linda, they sent me home *again!*"

"Any blood work? Any medications?" I asked. "Was there any contact with your surgeon?"

"No," Steve replied. "I went home again, and just got worse. I couldn't eat, and I got even more bloated. By this time, my sternum really hurt. My whole rib cage felt unsteady—like it might come apart!

"Then, one day Terry and I were watching TV and I started coughing really hard. I blew out about a pint of blood—out of my incision! And this thick custard-like stuff, too! Maybe it was closer to a quart! It filled a bath towel. And I didn't know what to do."

That was all Terry needed to gather Steve up in the car and ferry him immediately to Seattle, taking him directly to the surgeon's office. The staff there promptly recognized that something was desperately wrong, and rushed Steve by gurney to the adjoining hospital.

A quart of pus blowing out of Steve's chest? I knew that Steve had a knack for hyperbole; Steve called it "marketing." But even a teaspoon of pus leaking from a post-op CABG incision had a life-threatening implication: infection!

Steve was directly admitted to the hospital on September 16th—roughly two weeks after his surgery. He recounts a limbo period of several days where the surgeon would visit him a couple of times a day, pondering what to do. The nurses placed dressings the size of baby diapers over the chest incision; the dressings would fill with pus, and the nurses would change them.

Steve remembers his internist, Dr. Tauben, visiting him at least twice a day during this period. Steve overheard heated discussions in the background; the doctors were arguing about what to do next. Dr. Tauben insisted on bringing in an infectious disease specialist, and new antibiotics were started immediately. On September 29th, Steve was taken back to surgery for a second operation, this time to re-open his chest and drain out the pus.

"I woke up in the ICU," Steve recalled," with my sister Carole holding a picture of Brita on my chest. There were tubes everywhere—I think there were five tubes draining pus out of my chest, and a couple of machines that looked like radiators next to the bed."

Steve was referring to the drains, and the "chest tubes" that helped in the process of reinflating the lungs.

"I remember Dr. Tauben coming in twice a day—every single day. I remember the infectious disease doctor, Dr. Moss, so kind and so smart. He was really straight up with me. He said that it was a very serious infection. And at first, even after the pus was drained out, I didn't seem to be responding. But Dr. Moss said he hoped he could find the right combination of antibiotics for me.

"I knew it was serious, and I knew that they might not get a grip on the infection. I realized that I could die from this, but I also knew I had a chance. One of the oddest things was that while I was in the ICU, I watched the NYPD episode where Jimmy Smits' character *died* of exactly the same thing I had—an infection after heart surgery. They couldn't pull him out of it."

"Yikes," I said, "Great timing!"

"I guess I wasn't ready to be written out of *my* series," Steve quipped.

After about a week in the ICU, Steve was well enough to move to a private room, but this time, it was a spacious corner suite with a sweeping city and waterfront view—beautiful, really; I knew exactly the room he meant.

George and Cheryl brought four-year-old Brita in twice a day as Steve recovered. Drs. Tauben and Moss made regular visits at least every day. But Steve said the surgeon never came in; he never talked to Steve or any family or friends after the case.

"That hit me very hard," Steve said, "that this surgeon held my heart—cradled my heart in his hands—and probably saved my life. But then, I had no connection with him afterwards. What an intimate contact—he held my heart! The surgeon was so powerful, and I was so completely vulnerable. I just wonder if these guys even *get* it: they hold people's hearts in their hands three or four times a day!

"The most intimate of contact, with *no human intimacy at all!"*

Steve teared up, then covered his face with his hands and broke into sobs. "I used to be so tough, really strong. I could solve anything physically—that's all gone away. "I remember one day when I first went home after the CABG. I stood in the front of my bathroom mirror. There was transparent tape over my chest incision so I could see every suture. It looked like someone had hit me with an axe. All the bravado I had—all gone!"

As Steve and I talked, we cried and my big bear of a man let go of years of pent-up feelings of vulnerability, the frustration of having had a relatively routine operation go so terribly wrong.

When he surfaced, Steve asked, "So does all of that sound normal? I mean, to you as a doctor, does what happened to me sound like everything went the way it should have gone?"

"Well, Steve," I answered slowly, "you had a massive, life-threatening complication with a surgery that's done every day. You certainly could have died. But it doesn't mean that anything was necessarily *done* wrong. What do *you* think?"

"You mean, 'aside from *that,* Mrs. Lincoln, how did you like the play?'"

"Yeah, just like that! No seriously, is there anything *specific* that you think should have been done differently?"

"Well," Steve paused, "I would not go to that local ER again—ever. And I do believe that the X-ray technician there who lifted me onto that table injured my sternum. I heard a crack, and my sternum separated after that."

"Do you think that was intentional?"

"Oh, no. It was probably an accident, or maybe he did it out of ignorance."

"What about the surgeon?" I asked.

"I don't think he knew what to do when the real problems happened. He would come in and look at me, press on my moving sternum, and leave the room without a word. That was before the second surgery. I thought it was terrible that he never came to see me afterwards."

"Do you think it's possible you just don't remember him coming?

It sounds like you were pretty sick."

"It's possible, I guess," Steve answered, "but I do remember Dr. Moss and Dr. Tauben, and everyone else who came."

"Well, I have seen a dynamic where a doctor seems to 'check out' after something bad happens—a complication or a bad outcome. What I mean is, the doctor just stops communicating which, of course, is exactly the opposite of what you *should* do. I think when you have a complication, that's when you need to have the *most* visible presence. Let the patient know that you're in there working and trying to solve the problem!

"It certainly seems that Dr. Tauben and Dr. Moss were there for you. They went above and beyond—and probably saved your life."

"No doubt, Linda Jo. That was really impressive," Steve said.

He thought for a moment. "I guess when it's all said and done, I'm just glad to have made it through. But I am certain there was some controversy—at least some question—about how my case was managed.

"For my whole hospital stay—I mean for the second surgery—the ICU, the private suite, the home nursing care afterwards, and even for the six months of IV antibiotics when I went home—I never received a bill! *And I know that's unusual!"*

"Steve, all I can say is this: if you ever have surgery again, you know I will watch you like a hawk. And I'm a hell of an advocate—a mama lion. To the best of *my* ability, I would not let this happen to you again."

"I guess it could be different with a wife," he acknowledged.

"Steve, do you think you would ever have another bypass? After all that happened?" I asked.

He drew a deep breath. "To get a kidney? With a twelve-year-old? *You bet I would!"*

Several weeks after Steve's initial evaluation by the University of Washington transplant team, we received a matter-of-fact form letter. Dr. Somebody, the cardiologist, who had never met Steve and couldn't pick him out of a line-up, had decreed that Steve would be required to have another cardiac catheterization. Non-negotiable; no discussion. If Steve wanted a kidney, he would have to submit to the cardiac catheterization, with its one-in-five hundred to one-in-one thousand risk of a complication!

Chapter Twenty-Six

Steve arranged to have the required cardiac catheterization performed by his own cardiologist, Dr. Ali. On the morning of the procedure, the implications of the test weighed heavily on all of us. The best of all possibilities was that the study would show that the grafts from Steve's earlier bypass were still open, and that he had developed no new blockages requiring intervention such as a stent or another bypass. But eight-and-a-half years out from his last CABG (Coronary Artery Bypass Graft) with ongoing diabetes? This best-of-all-worlds' scenario seemed unlikely.

The second possibility was that Dr. Ali would discover new blockages that could be opened by means of coronary artery angioplasty. In angioplasty, a balloon is introduced via catheter into the narrowed coronary artery. The balloon is then inflated to compress the plaque against the vessel wall, widening the artery diameter. In such a procedure, a vessel could also be stented, i.e., a tiny coil could be introduced into the artery to buttress its walls open. The problem with these procedures, along with their inherent risks of complications, was the fact that Steve's kidney transplant could be put on hold *for another whole year!*

The third possibility was that the angiogram would show that Steve's heart disease had progressed to the point where he would need another

CABG. The very thought of another bypass brought back the horror of that unimaginable period in his life—the CABG with its overwhelming infection requiring a second surgery and six months of IV antibiotics afterwards. The horror of coming so close to losing everything, with a four-year-old daughter in the wings.

The last possibility, and always a possibility even with a routine cardiac catheterization, was that something would go wrong with the procedure itself: a stroke perhaps, a cardiac rhythm disturbance, even death.

So we waited and talked. I scratched Steve's shoulders. Steve had his chest shaved by a non-verbal little man with a Parkinsonian shuffle, and an IV was started by a cheerful nurse. And then, Steve was wheeled off for the cardiac cath with my good wishes and a kiss on the nose. I went to the hospital cafeteria to get some breakfast.

Probably an hour-and-a-half later, I ran into Dr. Ali in the hallway near the family waiting area.

"It's good news," she said. "The grafts look new, like they were just done!"

"And the rest of the vessels?" I asked.

"Maybe forty to fifty percent narrowing in some, but nothing we need to do anything about. It really looked good."

"That's the best news we could have gotten!" I said

Dr. Ali nodded.

"Now there *is* something I am concerned about. We got Steve's CBC back. His hematocrit is twenty-five, and his platelet count is only forty-four."

"That's new for him," I said. "His hematocrit has been running about twenty-eight, in spite of the Aranesp. And his platelets have been in the low-normal range, but never forty-four."

Dr. Ali said she'd talk with Dr. Thakur, Steve's nephrologist.

The hematocrit is the percentage of blood that is made up of red blood cells, the cells which carry oxygen to our tissues. In most humans, the blood is thirty-five to forty-five percent red cells; hence, the hematocrit runs between thirty-five and forty-five. Kidney patients have low hematocrits because their kidneys produce insufficient EPO, the kidney hormone that works on the bone marrow to stimulate red cell production. EPO can be given by injection (Aranesp is one brand of EPO), and as long as a person has adequate stores of iron, the bone marrow responds by producing new red blood cells. (We sometimes read of athletes using EPO illegally as a performance enhancer.) It was not clear if Steve was not making enough red cells, or if he was losing blood somehow.

The low platelet count was also worrisome. Like red cells, platelets are produced in the bone marrow. They are critical to our blood's clotting function, traveling to areas of injury to initiate a protective clot. I learned that the body can form antibodies to Heparin, an anticoagulant medication routinely used in dialysis. Such antibodies can attack and destroy platelets. We were relieved when a blood test proved that Steve did *not* have this antibody in his blood.

There was so much to learn! It seemed that Steve would dodge one bullet only to step into the cross-hairs of yet another enemy.

The day after Steve's cardiac catheterization, Dr. Thakur asked that Steve be evaluated by a hematologist, i.e., a blood specialist. I snatched up an appointment with an excellent hematology nurse practitioner for the same afternoon. The nurse practitioner was thorough and personable, and smart. I figured that a nurse practitioner specializing in hematology probably knew more about this field than most physicians. As always, I had to consider Steve's clinical situation along with our living situation. Tests that could be done seamlessly in Seattle were not available on Bainbridge Island. Plus, we were heading into Memorial Day weekend, when nothing medical would be done unless it was a clear emergency.

The nurse practitioner consulted with the hematologist; they recommended that Steve have a bone marrow biopsy to evaluate the condition of the bone marrow and to explore why it wasn't responding properly to the EPO and iron he was receiving. Anemia, after all, boils down to one of two problems; losing red cells or not producing enough of them.

A bone marrow biopsy would examine all three cell lines: red cells, white cells, and platelets. Steve was producing white cells in adequate numbers, but he was low in red cells and platelets. So while the infection-fighting capacity of the white cells was intact, the oxygen-carrying capacity of the red cells and the clotting capability of the platelets were both reduced.

In a bone marrow biopsy, a sample of marrow is harvested by plunging a six-inch trochar into the backside of the hip bone just below the waist. The marrow sample is then drawn out of the bone and into a syringe with two painful tugs. Plunging the needle into the bone requires considerable force. The trochar is actually anchored onto a thick square of wood to give the operator better traction; the device looks kind of like a corkscrew.

Steve agreed to the test, and the nurse practitioner was willing to do it right away. I was relieved; a test that takes several days for interpretation could have held Steve up, especially with the holiday weekend. Additionally Steve's hematocrit had fallen a full three points overnight (the equivalent of losing a unit of blood) even though there was no evidence of bleeding. Now twenty-two, would his hematocrit be fifteen by the weekend?

I hadn't done a bone marrow biopsy since residency. Now, I was observing one, with Steve lying on his stomach preparing for the pain. The nurse practitioner was remarkably smooth: all business but very kind. She harvested the sample with two swift pulls.

We headed back to the Island, awaiting the test results which would be available the next week.

Chapter Twenty-Seven

On Saturday, May 24th, I awoke to a resounding thud. Steve was lying face down, parallel to the bed.

"I fell," he murmured.

"How on earth did you fall?" I asked, as I jumped over the bed to look closer.

Steve looked dreadful, his skin pasty from his anemia. I could see that he had rug burns on his left forehead, his left shoulder, and on both knees and elbows. His eyes were watery from artificial tears and eye ointment; he looked dazed. Had he had a stroke? Was anything broken? With his low platelet count, could he be bleeding internally? Worse yet, could he have hit his head hard enough to be bleeding into his brain?

As I evaluated Steve, it seemed apparent that he was marginally okay; nothing catastrophic had occurred. It seemed that he had struck his left shoulder and rib cage, probably on the bed frame on the way down. The best Steve could figure was that he had stood up, half asleep, to relieve one of a dozen leg cramps he had had through the night. He then slipped on the sisal rug and went down hard.

Steve's medical fragility, and our overall vulnerability as a family, were becoming more apparent. If he had injured himself seriously, I wouldn't be able to pick him up. Steve outweighed me by over fifty pounds, and his strength and balance were so poor that he couldn't have helped himself up. All of a sudden, Steve looked older—even ten to twenty years older than his chronological age. I realized that his work was not physically demanding; most his consulting work was done by computer or phone, but how could he possibly conduct business of *any* kind in this increasingly weakened state? Was he soon to join the ranks of the fully disabled patients in the Kidney Center sub-basement?

I was envisioning my future with an uncharacteristic bleakness. Here I was with a seemingly eighty-year-old husband, and a twelve-year-old stepdaughter who liked me only intermittently. Was I to become a single parent once again?

The negatives of my circumstance loomed ahead: the drudgery of the Bainbridge Island commute, the stressful three-to-four-hour dialysis treatments five days a week. I had been keeping this schedule for only eight months—and there was no relief in sight.

The practices I had cultivated for my own mental health, specifically rowing and spinning, seemed so distant now. When I met Steve, I was rowing on Lake Union three mornings a week, spinning at least twice a week, and doing strength training. It wasn't uncommon for me to exercise twice a day. Now, twice a week was barely manageable.

I dreamed about rowing; one night I dreamt that I lost my boat—the twenty-seven-foot by twelve-inch shell that meant so much to me. I felt my body change, with muscle mass and strength fading and clothes fitting tighter. It wasn't a matter of laziness; I would have gladly traded the life-sucking commute for exercise. The dialysis, of course, was trickier: Steve would die without it.

I was sinking fast into a state of caregiver burn-out. The stress of managing Steve's dialysis, now with the enormous fistula needles, the ongoing precariousness of his diabetes with a recent blood sugar level dipping to a low of forty, and now this profound anemia. All of this would have been plenty for a full-time wife at home, with medical care easily accessible.

I developed a state of hypervigilence—always listening for his breathing, listening for nuances in his speech—any warning that signaled trouble ahead. I learned that we humans do not always rise to nobility in the face of adversity and exhaustion. Sometimes, we slink down into our old, dysfunctional coping patterns.

I countered Steve's crankiness with my own irritability. We fought bitterly; Steve was critical and I grew intolerant. We both found that fighting during dialysis was far too threatening. One time after Steve had asked if I had gone to medical school in Guatemala, I stormed out of the room stating, "You can finish your *own* damned dialysis!"

In reality, of course, I was so hard-wired as a caregiver that I would never conceive of leaving during a treatment! Indeed, I was every bit as much a prisoner of dialysis as Steve was. And my leaving, possibly due to my own genetic Catholicism, was simply not an option. We were both stuck, and it wouldn't be getting better any time soon.

I grew disgusted with Steve's physical state and his lack of attention to its impact on Brita and me. For example, Steve might whack his shin against the corner of the bed frame, and bleed freely from an open wound. His low platelet count would have contributed to the bleeding, and certainly he couldn't control that. But he'd just bleed and bleed without any apparent attempt to control it, dribbling blood on the new carpet and trashing our brand new bedroom.

Then, he developed a loose cough, productive of copious, rattling sputum. Like nothing else in medicine, I loathed sputum. It took me back to my early morning microbiology lab at the Veterans Administration Hospital. We'd have to prepare cultures of sputum from long-term smokers, cancer patients, and pneumonia patients every morning at eight a.m. sharp. And there was no sputum like VA sputum: mucoid, particulate, bloody, chunky, odiferous two-pack-a-day sputum—the one and only entity in medicine that threatened to put me over a basin! I grew repulsed by Steve's Fess Parker cough.

There were days when I realized I didn't even *like* Steve! I suspect that there are many caregivers who have similar feelings, but never speak of them. It was a sickening, trapped feeling, tangled up with guilt and self-doubt. How could I have *ever* gotten into this mess? With my marriage vows—and even more importantly, my vow never to harm Brita—I certainly couldn't, and wouldn't, get out.

Chapter Twenty-Eight

By Wednesday, May 29, 2008, Steve's hematocrit had dropped to twenty-two, and his platelet count was still low at forty-four. He received a blood transfusion that evening, and we caught the 1:35 a.m. ferry back to the Island. The next day—or more accurately, later the same day—we went to two appointments: one with the hematology team, and one with Steve's ophthalmologist, Dr. Cowen.

The hematology nurse practitioner and the hematologist both came to the appointment. The hematologist stood a slender five-foot-seven, by no means imposing in his *physical* presence. And while he seemed too young for the part, like Doogie Howser young, the academic credentials framed in the office boasted considerable expertise. The doctor sat with his back toward Steve and me, facing the computer screen as he spoke. I didn't know if this represented aloofness or superiority. It might have even signaled shyness. But it was hard for me *not* to interpret his body language as that of indifference.

The bone marrow biopsy had shown no clear explanation: there was a mild increase in the number of plasma cells, precursors to a type of white blood cells that make antibodies. In certain cases, an excess of plasma cells signals a blood malignancy called multiple myeloma. Steve "absolutely" did *not* have this, the hematologist explained with great authority.

But with all his knowledge and bravado, the expert hematologist said he simply didn't know why Steve was producing insufficient red cells and platelets.

"So what should I do?" Steve asked.

The hematologist reached over and literally *patted Steve on the head.*

"Just take the medications we give you and be a good patient!" he said.

I gasped! The doctor, I am certain, was just trying to be funny. But the attempt at humor backfired; this wasn't funny to us at all! Imagine: he patted my fifty-eight-year-old husband on the head with me—*a physician*—sitting right there. How would he treat a young woman patient?

The medicine that was suggested was an "empiric trial" of the anti-inflammatory steroid Decadron. When a physician suggests an empiric trial, he or she means that the treatment *might* help, and it probably won't hurt. But with high-dose steroids, an empiric trial could hurt. Steroids raise the blood sugar—a problem for a diabetic. Steroids can irritate the stomach lining, even to the point of causing ulcers. It was concerning, for example, to think of a bleeding ulcer in a man with few platelets to stop the bleeding. Steroids can cause temporary mental changes as well; I remember one patient with a full-blown steroid-induced psychosis hallucinating as she rocked on her knees in the hospital corridor. But, all in all, the empiric trial of steroids seemed reasonable. We had to do *something!*

After the hematology visit, we drove across town to see Dr. Cowen, Steve's ophthalmologist. Steve's vision had become blurry during the week prior—terrifying, as diabetes is a leading cause of blindness! Dr. Cowen felt the blurriness was due to an inflammation of the cornea, but when Steve's vision progressively worsened, he grew more concerned. We told him about the anemia and the low platelet count.

"I've seen something like this before," Dr. Cowen said. "It was in a woman with a severe vitamin deficiency related to alcohol. Do you drink?"

Steve shook his head, no.

"Well, I think this may be related to a vitamin deficiency. I don't think Steve has a group of separate problems here," he said, referring to the vision changes, the anemia, and the low platelet count.

"I think this is probably all related," he said. "All caused by one thing. You just haven't found it yet." Dr. Cowen sent us back to the hematologist with recommendations to draw vitamin levels from Steve's blood.

In medicine, I like to use a few old sayings with my patients. For instance, the saying "Common things commonly occur" implies that you are more likely to have a muscle tension headache than a brain tumor. Or the medical student favorite: "When you hear hoof beats, look for horses, not zebras!"

Unfortunately for Mr. Williams, he ran with horses and zebras alike. I did agree with Dr. Cowen, however. I felt there was likely to be a "unifying diagnosis," an explanation that tied the whole picture together.

We just hadn't found it yet.

Chapter Twenty-Nine

"Occam's Razor" is a term all medical students learn. It refers to the "single cut," one simple explanation for a variety of symptoms. As the saying went, you *could* have "lice and fleas," i.e., two completely separate diseases occurring together. But it was always more compelling, and usually more realistic, to tie separate symptoms together under a common diagnostic umbrella.

By the middle of June 2008, Steve with his low hematocrit and low platelet count had received three units of blood to boost the red cell count. He had also received a course of Decadron, an anti-inflammatory steroid, to bolster his platelet production. It seemed that both levels were increasing, and Steve's cloudy vision was beginning to improve as well.

But no one, including the celebrated hematologist, could explain the unexpected constellation of symptoms. Steve and I decided to seek a second opinion from another hematologist. I think most good doctors welcome second opinions. I tell my own patients that the only time *not* to get a second opinion is when it delays urgent treatment, and the patient loses valuable time.

We met Dr. Sam Tolman on Monday, June 20th. In many ways, Sam was the antithesis of the first hematologist. Rather than being arrogant and dismissive, Sam was friendly and inclusive. He discussed concepts with open equivocation—thinking out loud as he discussed Steve's predicament.

When he spoke to me, Sam spoke in "medicine"; when he spoke to Steve, he broke things down a bit more, always making sure Steve understood. He was never condescending to either of us. With open eyes and steady listening skills, Sam was a communicator. He seemed kind. And there was nothing lacking in Sam's credentials; he just didn't choose to advertise them.

Sam, like Smiley, was concerned that Steve had multiple myeloma, a malignancy affecting the plasma cells of the bone marrow. The cellular components of our blood, i.e., red cells, white cells, and platelets, are all made deep within the spongy tissue of the bones—the marrow. And plasma cells are a type of white cell precursors. These are the cells that will become antibody-forming "B-lymphocytes," white cells which are critical to our body's immune function.

"So it looks like you may have myeloma," Sam began.

He reviewed the anemia, the low platelet count, and Steve's history of "MGUS" (monoclonal gammopathy of undetermined significance—pronounced "em-gus"). MGUS is a fairly common condition where plasma cells make abnormal proteins. In most cases MGUS causes no problems at all; but in others, MGUS can progress into multiple myeloma.

"But I thought the bone marrow biopsy showed *no* myeloma," I protested. "Seven-and-a-half percent plasma cells—that's what we heard from the other hematologist. Here—I have the report."

"I know," sighed Sam, "but it may depend on the sample location. You may find more plasma cells in another spot."

We were to learn that multiple myeloma consists of a hodge-podge of diagnostic criteria that resembles a Chinese restaurant menu: one criterion from Column A plus one criterion from Column B—or three criteria from Column B. Column A represented "major criteria" and Column B represented "minor criteria."

Thirty percent plasma cells in the marrow, for example, was a major criterion. When the bone marrow was crowded by abnormal plasma cells, the normal cells didn't have room to mature. This could well have explained Steve's lack of platelets and his low red cell count. Elevated levels of specific proteins produced by abnormal plasma cells, or a bone biopsy showing an isolated tumor of plasma cells were the two other "major criteria." Steve had none of these.

Minor criteria included a bone marrow biopsy showing ten to thirty percent plasma cells, a lower-than-normal level of antibodies, and an abnormal "skeletal survey." A skeletal survey is a collection of X-rays done to evaluate the skull, spine, hips, and long bones of the arms and legs. The survey tracks characteristic "lytic lesions" in the bones, places where the bones were eroded from the inside by the abnormal plasma cells. The skull, for example, would have a typical "punched out" appearance—round holes eaten into the bone from the inside. One of myeloma's most sinister effects was the thinning of long bones, sometimes leading to fractures. Steve likened the condition to being eaten alive—from the inside out—a horrifying image.

There was also a relationship between multiple myeloma and renal failure though nobody thought Steve's renal failure was myeloma-induced. Still, the triple threat of diabetes, renal failure, and a brewing myeloma brought new concerns for Steve's treatment and prognosis.

It is important to point out that while there does exist a continuum linking MGUS with multiple myeloma, MGUS is usually benign. There are also definitions of "indolent myeloma," and "smoldering myeloma," making things even more bewildering. Multiple myeloma is highly variable, and can take years to diagnose.

Sam explained that multiple myeloma was treatable with medication, i.e., chemotherapy, and in some cases with radiation or stem cell transplants. But multiple myeloma—at the time—was not considered curable. Therapies would buy time and improve quality of life. But ultimately, remissions would end and a person would die of the disease as the bone marrow failed to produce normal cells.

To make things worse, not all of the treatments would be available to a patient with renal failure. Stem cell transplants, for example, would be far too risky. And at least one of the available drugs would likely worsen peripheral neuropathy—the numbness and pain in the feet. Worsening neuropathy could increase Steve's risks for falls and fractures. Myeloma itself carried an increased risk of fractures due to bone weakening and erosion.

What a circuitous nightmare! Each of Steve's several medical conditions could play on his other medical problems, either by directly making them worse or by eliminating available treatment options.

"There is another concern," explained Dr. Tolman.

Steve and I looked worried.

"If Steve does have multiple myeloma—and remember we don't know for certain that he does, but if Steve has multiple myeloma, *he will no longer be eligible for a kidney transplant."*

This giant "other shoe," no kidney transplant, hit with a reverberating thud. No kidney transplant significantly reduced Steve's statistical longevity, i.e., his "virtual" lifespan. Twenty years shrunk to eight years for a "healthy" patient with End Stage Renal Disease. My reading on multiple myeloma projected a life span of two to five years—and that was in the "healthy" myeloma patient! Steve would be neither a healthy kidney patient, nor a healthy myeloma patient.

If a person had another potentially terminal disease, a donated kidney would be more responsibly used in a more "viable" candidate. A donor kidney had to be reserved for someone who was expected to live longer. Additionally, kidney transplants always required the use of industrial-grade anti-rejection drugs. These drugs suppress the immune system to help the transplanted kidney survive, but also increase the patient's risk of other malignancies: lymphoma, skin cancers, colon cancer, and others.

"So no kidney transplant" said Steve. "So I'm basically fucked."

"Well, remember if you do have myeloma, there is a lot we can do to treat it and prevent its complications," said Dr. Tolman.

"But you can't cure it," said Steve.

"That's true," said Dr. Tolman. "But, you know, Steve, a kidney transplant is not without its *own* risks. And we have some very promising new drugs which are well tolerated by patients."

"And then there's nocturnal dialysis, Steve," I chimed in. "We've read that nocturnal dialysis can be almost as good as a transplant—at least far better than regular dialysis—both in keeping you alive and in helping you feel better."

Dr. Tolman suggested that Steve obtain a skeletal survey to evaluate his bones, and recommended a follow-up bone marrow biopsy as well.

Steve looked devastated. "No transplant" was a tough pill to swallow.

Our world shifted again. The threat of multiple myeloma appeared grimly ahead, and "mere" End Stage Renal Disease didn't look so ominous to us anymore.

Chapter Thirty

The nurse from the first hematologist's office phoned Steve to reschedule his cancelled appointment. She made a point of emphasizing that the *doctor* wanted to see Steve. Steve scheduled the appointment over my disapproving sigh. I railed against the superiority of the first doctor, and I had bonded instantly with Dr. Tolman.

"I need the best information out there, Linda Jo," said Steve. "And I don't care if the guy who delivers it is a total jerk. I don't need the information sugar-coated. Besides, don't you think reputation counts?"

"Of course it counts," I snapped, "but so does being involved. So does being kind. This new guy may actually *care* about your outcome. He may work harder for you than the other guy. And these doctors don't work in a vacuum. They have tumor boards to review cases."

"Well, why do you think he's asking me to come in?" asked Steve, referring to the first hematologist. "Maybe he's reviewed my numbers. Maybe he is going to tell me *now* that I have multiple myeloma."

"Maybe so, " I said. "I don't know. Why don't you just make the appointment and see what he has to say. But schedule the skeletal survey too."

Over the next few days, Steve had the skeletal survey completed: X-rays of his arms, legs, hips, spine, and skull. I had the report faxed directly to me at my medical office. There were several areas of boney abnormalities "compatible with myeloma."

Another blow! I knew radiologists well enough to know that they equivocate for a living. They write general qualifiers like: "neoplasm cannot be excluded," or "clinical correlation recommended." Both of these mean, "It could be this awful diagnosis, but then again, maybe not! You decide!"

A radiologist friend of mine used to tell the joke:

Q: What is the favorite food of the radiologist?

A: Waffles.

But here it was in Steve's report: three specific areas of boney abnormality which were "compatible with myeloma." Period. No "*may be* compatible with myeloma." No "clinical correlation suggested." Granted, an abnormal skeletal survey was considered a minor criterion for multiple myeloma, but it seemed awfully major to me.

So the next week, Steve and I went back to see the first hematologist: going to get the tablets from the mountain. Going to see what wisdom this top-rated hematologist had to offer.

"So, where are we?" the specialist began. "Have we done a bone marrow on you yet?"

Christ, have we done a bone marrow? I thought. *Where have you been all this time?*

"Yes, here it is," he said, reading the report. "So, it has some features of multiple myeloma, but it isn't definitive.

"And then," he continued, "we did a skeletal survey."

You did not, you arrogant son-of-a-bitch! The other doctor tumbled to that idea!

I handed him the computer DVD with the skeletal survey, and he loaded it into his computer. The logo from the *other* hospital screamed out our medical infidelity, but the specialist didn't seem to notice.

"So it has some areas of concern," he pondered. "Again, not definitive."

"What about Steve's UPEP?" I asked, referring to a twenty-four-hour urine collection aimed at identifying abnormal proteins.

The hematologist fumbled through Steve's chart—admittedly, the size of the Seattle telephone directory. "I can't find it," he said with irritation. "I'll have the lab fax it to me. That should clinch the diagnosis."

He left the room, and Steve and I could hear a flurry of activity as staff members flew into action to find the missing test result. A copy arrived from the lab a full hour later. But by that time, I had located it myself, deep in the bowels of Steve's medical file—and it was *abnormal!* I was seething!

The doctor entered the room.

"So the UPEP (urine protein electrophoresis) is abnormal," he said.

"Does Steve have multiple myeloma?" I asked.

"I don't know," he paused. "I don't want to say you have it if the situation is really ambiguous. That would take you out of the transplant program."

"So what should we do?" Steve asked.

The hematologist folded his arms across his chest and stroked his chin. "Well, you are a complicated patient, Mr. Williams," he began, "and in your case, I think you should go to the Hutch and get an opinion from them."

The "Hutch" was the old name for Seattle's premier cancer center, now combining the resources of the University of Washington, the old Fred Hutchinson Cancer Research Center, and Children's Hospital. And the recommendation to seek their opinion was quite reasonable, although it may have represented a bit of a defeat for the brilliant young hematologist.

None of this mattered to me. I was fuming as we took the information and left the office. Perhaps it was the compounded anger and frustration I had accumulated during the months of Steve's illness. Perhaps it was because I so despise arrogance in medicine. Perhaps I was so enraged because this arrogant expert—whom Steve had trusted—had built up Steve's hope for information and came to our critical meeting *with his pants down!* He was inadequately prepared, and no amount of experience or credentialing could negate that fact!

We walked slowly to the car, and sat quietly for a while.

"What do you think?" I asked, reaching for Steve's hand.

"Well, he was clearly unprepared," Steve replied. "He didn't have any new information at all. And I am seriously fucked here."

"Maybe the information isn't *knowable* yet, Steve," I offered. "Sometimes it takes a while for the full information to unfold. I am so terribly disappointed. Maybe he just doesn't want to label you with a diagnosis and ace you out of a transplant. Do you want to go to the Hutch for another opinion?"

"I want to talk to the expert. I want to talk to Dr. Myeloma. I don't want to jump on any rush to a diagnosis. You, Smiley, and Tolman all have me having multiple myeloma."

"I don't *want* you to have myeloma, Steve. But if you do have it, I want you to be treated so you can live as long as possible and as well as possible. You know—no fractures, no complications that we could have prevented.

"Besides," I continued, "we've got this dialysis thing *down* now. And with nocturnal dialysis, you will be feeling better. I will do dialysis on you for the rest of my life. I don't care."

So again, End Stage Renal Disease paled in importance: an anemic little dragon that we knew how to *manage*.

Chapter Thirty-One

That evening, Steve and I went to a movie, *The Visitor,* a beautiful little film about an emotionally empty professor whose world was opened by an unlikely set of foreigners squatting in his extra apartment. Huddled close to Steve, I watched a hopeful couple stroll across the screen. Steve never strolled. We would never *stroll* together—ever.

I started to cry, silently sobbing in the movie, tears coming too fast to catch. We finished the beautiful film and limped back to the car. On our way home, and in bed that night, I cried. We both cried. The fears, the frustrations, the anger, the anticipatory sorrow all tumbled out.

"I'm sorry, Linda Jo. I'm so sorry."

"Sorry for what?" I sniffled. "You have nothing to apologize for."

"I am sorry to put you through this hell."

"You would never have chosen this, Stephen. I know that."

We kept on crying, each new thought bringing up a new reason to cry. Brita, especially: how could we help her through *this?* How do you pluck the sun out of a child's universe and expect her to survive intact? What about our work, our friends, our family?

How could it be that we each had just found love: rich, compatible love—only to see it ridiculed by the assembling dragons?

"We only just found each other!" I sobbed. "Nobody has ever loved me as much as you do! And I'm not that easy to love! What do you think I would do without you? Kayak? Do you think that would be enough? And how could I raise Brita without you? I don't want to be a single parent again!"

"I love you a fucking ton, Linda Jo," Steve sniffled. "The only things I have ever cared about are you and Brita. Nothing else. Nothing else."

We cried into the night until we both succumbed to sleep. We had gathered all the questions. We would work on the answers later.

Chapter Thirty-Two

During early July 2008, we welcomed a bit of a reprieve. The weather converted our gray "January" into a carefree balmy July. Even the ferry rides were beautiful, with our boats heading into brilliant evening sunsets. No new medical bulletins had arisen. We were getting into the rhythm of night-time dialysis. The new style required runs of seven hours every other night, as opposed to three-hour runs five days a week. It still took an hour to get Steve hooked up to the machine, but it felt more like "tucking him in" at night than performing a medical procedure. At least I could frame it that way. The theory was that extended dialysis done more slowly over a longer period of time was more effective in clearing toxins.

The dialysis nights were tricky for me because I had to get out of bed to respond to a couple of expected alarm signals, and then unhook Steve from the machine at the end of the run. There could be other alarm signals also—potentially serious alarms which required trouble-shooting.

It meant interrupted sleep for me, and to a lesser extent for Steve. But because it freed up our early evenings, I was able to get back to regular strength training and spinning classes. I even went kayaking and rowing, with each event reminding me that I was still the same person—a few pounds heavier perhaps, but still the same person.

Steve's color began to improve. He felt more energetic and less "foggy." He noticed an improvement in his peripheral neuropathy symptoms, and his gait grew steadier. Food began to taste better, and his appetite picked up.

For brief moments, we could forget about the health nightmares, and carry on with our routines. Our focus shifted to getting Brita off to Dolphin Camp—a week-long Florida adventure with her science class. We turned our attention to selling our homes; like so many others, we were caught up in the real estate crisis and were feeling its financial strain. We had purchased the condo cottage before selling Steve's beautiful home, and now carried two mortgages. We had to stop the financial bleeding; it was an engrossing necessity. A niece had eloped unexpectedly, and announced her pregnancy; the family was adjusting to the news. And, of course, we had our work, all of which would have been fully occupying without the kidney dialysis or the greater worry of multiple myeloma.

During the reprieve, however, we savored that delicious glimpse of life without the burden of apparent mortality—at least no immediate threats. Of course, we all live with the dulled understanding that natural disasters, automobile accidents, and those occasional out-of-the-blue heart attacks do happen. But during a reprieve, these things happen to *other* people. We welcomed, relished, the perceived return to normalcy.

Chapter Thirty-Three

At the end of July 2008, Brita went off to Dolphin Camp in Florida for a week of "science," interspersed with swimming with dolphins, gator-watching, and other summer activities, which required a bikini. It would be a grand adventure for Brita, already a world traveler. And Steve and I could devote a few evenings to one of his passions—catching the latest newly released films. (How could anyone possibly rest with the new *Batman* in town?)

On Friday of that week, Steve and I were to attend the sixtieth birthday party of David Graebener, a long-time friend and business partner from the audio industry. Steve had one detail to complete before the party. Dr. Tolman, Steve's new hematologist, had recommended a trial of "WinRho," an intravenous medication that would help us figure out whether Steve really did have multiple myeloma, or a much less worrisome platelet disorder called "ITP" (idiopathic thrombocytopenic purpura). In ITP, platelets are gobbled up by the spleen, resulting in lower-than-normal platelet counts. If Steve really did have ITP, the WinRho would block the destruction of the platelets, and the platelet count would rise. WinRho, however, wouldn't touch multiple myeloma.

Steve completed the IV drip, and left the Medical Treatment Center to proceed with his Friday afternoon errands. Suddenly, however, his body began to shake violently, almost convulsively. Then came hot sweats and icy chills, and waves of the famous Steve Williams' nausea following close behind. In the midst of Aurora Avenue, a major arterial, Steve made an illegal U-turn and rushed back to the Medical Treatment Center.

"I'm coming apart at the seams, Linda Jo. I don't know what's wrong," Steve explained to me over the cell phone.

"Sounds like a reaction to the medication, Steve. Are you breathing okay?"

"Yes, but I'm shaking so hard, I can barely drive. I'm almost there."

"Well, get there as fast as you can, but stay on the phone with me."

That was probably not the best advice for someone having an acute reaction; Medic One would have been a more prudent suggestion. Sometimes, though, just getting to the facility *fast* is the best course.

Steve made it to the hospital; I could hear him talking to the nurses on my cell phone. Then, I could hear him gagging and vomiting, howling like a wounded animal.

By the time I arrived, the nurses had administered IV Benadryl, an antihistamine, and Tylenol to reduce Steve's climbing fever. Steve's vomiting had started in earnest, with Steve filling every receptacle available.

"I have to go to the bathroom," Steve announced. "I mean *right now!"*

The nurse and I helped Steve to the toilet, but the overwhelming volume of diarrhea was too much to control. I cleaned Steve up with a wet washcloth, and stuffed his soiled clothing into a plastic hospital bag.

"He will be more comfortable in these," said the nurse, handing me a giant pair of adult "Pull-Ups."

We tugged the "Executive Underjams" into position; not a picture I would have imagined from our Match.com days, but in every respect a picture of true intimacy.

But when Steve began having pressure across the front of his chest, it was time to move to the hospital Emergency Room. I knew his recent cardiac catheterization had given reassuring information about Steve's cardiac status, but who knew? Certainly, Steve could be having ischemic chest pain—perhaps a heart attack.

In the ER Steve's EKG was unchanged from his normal, but his white blood cell count rocketed from a normal 5000 to 24,000! Steve was pouring out infection-fighting white cells. Were we on the right track? Could Steve really be having an acute onset of sepsis—bacteria in the bloodstream? As a diabetic, he was at greater risk for developing sepsis than the average person.

The rest of Steve's lab work, however, supported a reaction to the medication: his liver enzymes soared, with a bilirubin of 4.7 mg/deciliter (normal being about 1.0). Steve's cardiac enzymes (CK-MB and troponin) shot up as well. It was a confusing picture, but nobody had any question that Steve needed to stay the night. We all tucked him into a telemetry bed, where Steve's heart rhythms could be monitored overnight; I assembled yet another lumpy hospital cot for myself.

By the next morning, Steve felt marginally better, but his urine was the color of cola. The dark urine reflected the pigment from broken red blood cells, characteristic of a hemolytic anemia. The reaction to the WinRho was causing Steve's red blood cells to "lyse" or break (hence, the term "hemolytic"). The on-call hematologist felt that Steve's reaction might take several days to run its course.

Little by little, Steve's labs normalized, though his red cell count and his hematocrit dropped in response to the red cell destruction. His urine transitioned from the color of cola to tea, and it was established that he had not suffered a heart attack. But the platelet count hovered under sixty. Multiple myeloma was still strongly in the running.

By Monday of that week, Brita was scheduled to return from the dolphins. We had not been to David's party; we had not seen *Batman*. We dispatched Tim to pick up Brita from the airport; the information that Steve was in the hospital had sent her to the shower in tears. We hadn't included Brita in the blow-by-blow myeloma saga because the diagnosis wasn't certain. What do you do, after all? Send a kid to Dolphin Camp with "Have fun; we think your dad may have blood cancer?" We thought not. Naturally, Brita would receive full disclosure when we knew—really knew—her dad's diagnosis.

Chapter Thirty-Four

Still no answers. Steve's reaction to WinRho was severe, but it could have happened to anyone, and it didn't imply anything other than another "bit" of bad luck. Steve needed another bone marrow biopsy to determine the types of cells his bone marrow was making. An increase in plasma cells to over ten percent would add another "minor criterion" for myeloma (he already had two—the abnormal skeletal survey and the MGUS). Certainly, a finding of thirty percent plasma cells would cement the diagnosis altogether.

Resigned to our fate, Steve and I prepared for the bone marrow biopsy appointment with Dr. Tolman. Sucking marrow from a hip bone, and boring out a core of bone to study couldn't possibly be painless. Steve described it as "lively," but also said that Sam's procedure was the least painful of the marrow collections he'd experienced.

We returned to the Cancer Center the next week, sitting in the waiting room with another collection of folks who had shared, in some way, a common history. The magazines in this waiting room seemed to be mostly cancer-focused; what else mattered? A large wicker basket offered hand-knit stocking caps to shelter balding chemotherapy heads from the Northwest chill; a couple of jars held wrapped hard candies for dry chemotherapy mouths. And there were giant jigsaw puzzles on game tables to occupy people's time and minds.

The Cancer Center waiting room contained a wide age range of folks, although some of the younger people were there with parents. There were of course, hairless people, people waiting for chemotherapy treatments, frightened-looking people (like us), and robust, triumphant people who had either done well or were doing well in "bucking up."

One genderless person breezed by on a stretcher, gaunt and bald, with a gaze locked on the ceiling. It's a curious thing about diagnosis-specific waiting rooms. Clearly, we see people with cancer—or kidney failure—all around us in the world; it's just that we see them diluted by the general population. In the Cancer Center, the cancer patients reached a critical mass: a share too large to ignore, an in-your-face diagnosis that couldn't be denied. I learned long ago in medicine: the most together-appearing people can harbor the most unimaginable pain. You simply never know what burdens people carry.

Steve's name was called, and we shuffled back to Dr. Tolman's exam to get the bone marrow results.

Hit us again, I thought, *hit us again.*

Sam began by reviewing the lab results from blood drawn earlier that day. Steve's hematocrit was a respectable thirty-three percent, reflecting the transfusion he had received a few days before. The platelet count was one-hundred-thirty, still relatively high from the steroids he'd been given in the hospital.

"What about the marrow?" I asked.

"The bone marrow is *normal,*" Sam said.

We all stopped to breathe. "Normal" was a word that rarely involved Steve Williams, actually in *any* context.

"What do you mean . . . normal?" I asked.

"Steve has two percent plasma cells," explained Dr. Tolman. "So he doesn't have either a major or minor criteria for myeloma on the basis of this marrow biopsy.

"Steve's marrow actually shows excellent reserve. He's making plenty of healthy new cells, and in the right proportions. It would be just the opposite in cancer."

Steve and I just looked at each other. This was completely unexpected.

We were stumped by the good news, neither of us knowing how to react.

"So," continued Sam, "I can't say that Steve has multiple myeloma. He does have the MGUS, so he will always be at some risk to *get* multiple myeloma someday. But he doesn't have it now.

"How do we account for the low platelets, then?" I asked.

"I think we'll have to call it an atypical ITP. And it may be simply the result of his dialysis. It's not common, but it is something we can monitor. We know that Steve is very responsive to steroids, so we can treat him with steroids if needed."

"So, the anemia may have been simply due to iron deficiency. And, of course, the renal failure," I said.

Sam nodded.

"What about the skeletal survey?" I pressed.

"Hard to say," Sam began. "But you remember, a skeletal survey isn't definite.

"At this point, we may want to pursue a bone biopsy in one of the areas that looked abnormal. We may want to try to *prove* that Steve does not have multiple myeloma. Then, we can send him back to the kidney transplant team at the University of Washington; he may be a transplant candidate again."

He may be a transplant candidate again! He may be a candidate for the potent anti-rejection drugs, for the risk of other cancers. He may be a candidate for that major, life-threatening surgery, and the treacherous wait for that compatible kidney.

But he might be a candidate for that *twenty-year* life span! We sat in disbelief, struggling to assimilate the promising news. We had both become so guarded, so protective. It was difficult to let in news that might actually be good.

That night, Steve and I watched *Hopkins,* a medical program on TV. In one of its segments, the program portrayed a three-couple kidney transplant swap. They showed the actual surgery, with a freshly transplanted kidney just connected to the recipient's blood vessels. After a moment or two, the new kidney began to produce steady drops of urine. The transplanted kidney was going to work—in a woman who had endured years of chronic kidney failure and dialysis, and now awaited the arrival of her first grandbaby with the promise of a more normal life!

"That never gets old," commented the transplant surgeon as he watched the urine drip from the newly created site.

No, I thought, *I imagine hope never gets old.*

We would see Dr. Thakur again in another week or so, and talk to him about the possibility of kidney transplant once again. And Steve would make arrangements for an MRI and bone biopsy to prove—once and for all—that multiple myeloma was a non-issue.

The shoulder MRI, performed in August 2008, was medically unremarkable—nothing damning. The next step was a whole-body PET scan. In a PET scan, labeled glucose molecules are injected into the bloodstream. The labeled glucose molecules then move to areas that are "metabolically active," i.e., areas which require more energy. A cancer, for example, is highly active—using more energy than other cells. Thus, cancerous areas "light up" on a PET scan as they soak up more of the labeled glucose to use for energy.

Steve's PET scan, like the MRI, showed nothing remarkable. Dr. Tolman felt that the final proof would require taking an actual bone specimen from one of the areas which seemed suspicious on the original skeletal survey; in this case, the thigh bone. The procedure was done under local anesthesia: hammers and chisels auguring into the firm bone to harvest three generous chips of bone.

Steve's femur bone and quadriceps muscle ached for days after the sampling. But the results justified the pain: "No abnormal B- or T-cell population, no abnormal plasma cell population . . . no plasma cell neoplasm is identified."

In other words, no multiple myeloma. The MGUS (monoclonal gammopathy of uncertain significance) would not disappear, and it could progress to myeloma at some point.

Steve's anemia was attributed to both his kidney failure (decreased EPO) and iron deficiency, and the low platelets were finally labeled an "atypical ITP," "idiopathic thrombocytopenia," which translated to "low platelets, and we don't really know why."

We never did find that unifying diagnosis that included Steve's vision changes, but his vision improved. We attributed the problem to nutritional deficiencies. Steve had, after all, cut back drastically on his food intake. It was a vicious circle: he'd feel so poorly, he wouldn't eat. Then, he'd feel worse, and so on. It had been a roller coaster ride of medical minutiae.

Ironically, the first hematologist, against whom I'd railed in fury and frustration, turned out to be correct about Steve's not having multiple myeloma. He was also on the money with the empiric trial of Decadron to increase Steve's platelet count. I recalled my residency adage, "If you're going to be arrogant, you'd better be right." He *was* right, and that fact bears acknowledgement.

It was the best news possible in our challenging situation. We were going to go back to the University of Washington Transplant Program, and back to the business of finding a compatible kidney.

Chapter Thirty-Five

On August 16, 2008, Steve celebrated his fifty-ninth birthday with a party that sister Carole hosted on the roof deck of her Pike Place Market condominium. How normal it seemed to see Steve standing at the barbecue—wearing his summer uniform of a stained T-shirt and saggy jeans—flipping burgers and sausages, grilling chicken. He was in his glory, with good friends, good food, and the promise of a future restored.

As we served up the birthday apple pie, Steve and I reminisced over the year. Steve looked and felt far better than he did at his previous birthday—thinner perhaps, certainly not carrying the bloat of the impending renal failure, and decidedly more relaxed. What an arduous year it had been!

As August moved on, our family readied Brita for her start at her new middle school. Our attention turned to schedules, soccer, and the mundane routine of buying school supplies.

The "cues" from the universe, e.g., the color of the sky, the change in ambient light, and the standard events of starting a new school year brought what is known in medicine as the "Anniversary Phenomenon," that visceral, even subconscious recognition of a time of previous grief or vulnerability.

We had come full circle: back to the season in which Steve began his free-fall into kidney hell. *This* fall, however, our focus would be getting Stephen on "the list" to receive a cadaveric kidney for transplant; perhaps we could even find a living donor—a compassionate friend who was willing to step up to give Steve that ultimate gift. Like all families impacted by End Stage Renal Disease, we would live our lives tethered to dialysis … but we would get to live the lives we had.

Chapter Thirty-Six

So, what had we learned through this important year? We learned, of course, a boatload of detail about diabetes and renal failure. Now, when my own patients take their diabetes less seriously than would be optimal, I point to Steve's example. This disease has more complications than one might imagine. It must be prevented when possible, and treated aggressively when identified. The renal complications of diabetes are life-changing, particularly when culminating in End Stage Renal Disease. Patients must know about these complications; they do happen to real people. And I feel patients must know about the simple blood tests which are available to monitor their progress (eGFR or estimated glomerular filtration rate; now available on many standard blood screens).

We learned, faced with End Stage Renal Disease, that we could master the elegant technology of home dialysis. Compassionate, well-informed dialysis nurses were there to teach us and guide us. We could regain some control over the disease by taking its management into our own hands.

We learned intimately of the subcultures of people with various diseases. There are whole groups of seemingly anonymous people who suffer in ways specific to their disease, but who work, play, and make the most of the lives they have. We appreciated that such groups are instrumental in helping individuals take control of their lives by sharing practical information, educating others about treatment options, and by providing examples to prove that life does go on.

We learned that organ transplantation represents a gift of technology, which provides unsurpassed hope for people with kidney failure. *All* individuals should talk with their loved ones about their own status as potential organ donors, and consider checking the organ donor box when renewing a driver's license.

We learned that when people say, "It couldn't possibly get any worse," that it *can* get worse! Steve and I would say, "At least it's not the burn unit!" And, always, the very worst would be one of our *children* in the burn unit.

We also learned, however, that when it did get worse from time to time, we did handle it. We noticed, however, that we were more likely to revert to old coping patterns than to rise to nobility. But somehow, somewhere, resources would surface. We managed; we survived, with new gratitude and a new appreciation for the love of a partner and an implausible new family.

We learned that a life-threatening chronic illness impacts *all* members of the family—not just the patient. Brita, for example, was shortchanged by parents who necessarily focused on keeping Dad alive, but didn't have the physical energy to get up in the early morning to see her off to school. Was this a reasonable trade-off? In the end, of course it was; it simply had to be that way. We would acknowledge it as a required, but poignant exchange. It just made us sad.

We learned, though it was no bulletin to me, that medicine is complicated. There aren't always clear explanations; we don't have all the answers. I've often told my patients when struggling with a problem, "This is medicine, not accounting!"

We learned that it can be totally reasonable to seek a second medical opinion, even if the issue is a nebulous matter of personal style. Unless getting that second opinion delays critical care for you or your loved one, seek it out. Good doctors welcome second opinions.

As for myself, I learned that being the primary caregiver, with home dialysis or any other chronic illness, requires attention to the most basic elements of *self* care: healthy food, vigorous exercise, maintaining friendships as one can, looking for humor, and nurturing anything which feeds the heart and soul. Ironically for me, "that fucking boat" ultimately provided stolen time and a refuge for writing our story. Left to my own devices, I might have time-managed around it, never benefiting from the personal therapy of writing this journal. It is my deepest hope that this story will help someone else who is engaged in a similar battle, underscore the value of organ transplantation, and maybe—just maybe—help some other soul *avoid* preventable kidney failure.

I learned much as a physician: our word choices, our posture, our body language all count so much in helping people through the challenges of their lives. *Being prepared* for a patient's appointment is critical; being respectful counts! We were fortunate to have worked with the likes of Drs. Thakur, Ali, and Tolman, and all of the other extremely kind health care providers who assisted us. As doctors, we never know the burdens our patients carry, but we do have real skills to help our patients shoulder them.

Finally, I was reminded that our personal encouragement and guidance come from everywhere: that gut feeling, the "happenstance" meeting with someone important in shaping a pivotal time, a dream, an audible message when there's no one around, or even the gift of an unexpected inheritance that somehow shows us our way. As we *pay attention,* we do receive guidance. In receiving, we are reminded to "pay it forward," and offer our hearts to the next traveler along the road.

The End

Acknowledgements

We extend our heartfelt thanks to the staff and volunteers of the Northwest Kidney Centers—the organization that gave us the tools to live as a family in the face of End Stage Renal Disease.

Our most sincere thanks are extended to the following individuals who have played a special part in this story. Although some are not specifically named in the book, they have clearly contributed to our experience in practical and positive ways. Our apologies to anyone who has been inadvertently omitted.

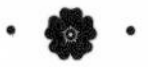

Humera Ali, MD
Melinda Archide, RN
Dan Ashcraft
Barbara Boni
Bob Bost
Donald A. Cornell
JoAnn B. Cornell
Sheldon Cowen, MD
Jim Croft
Terry and Penny Donofrio
Mary Dooley, MSW
Andrew M. Faulk, MD
Linda Franklin
Timothy Gromko Franklin
Erika Goldstein, MD
David Graebener
Florence Gromko
Don Gronachan
Richard L. Hagen
Jean Hutton, RN
Robert Jaffe, MD
Jean Kusumi, RN
Tom Martin
George and Cheryl Mead
Bonnie and Alan Mearns
Randi Mezich
Donna Mitchell
Steven R. Mitchell, MD PhD

Anthony Moore
Gregory Moss, MD
Robert Ness
Rex Ochi, MD
Janis Omri, RN
Hannah Peters
Carol Pettes, RN
Michael and Andrea Ramage
Sarah Rassa, RN
Neves Rigodanzo-Massey, RN
Steve and Mary Robertson
Cornelius Rosse MD
Larry and Dixie Running
Ben Shepherd
Roy and Cindy Simonson
Connie Jo Smith, MD
Suzi Spinner
Bruce Stanley
David Tauben, MD
S. Smiley Thakur, MD
Samuel Tolman, MD
James Watson, MD
James K. Weber MD
Brita Williams
Carole Jo Williams
Bessie Young, MD

Special gratitude is extended to my very patient editor and Literary Midwife, Elizabeth Lyon.

Order Form

To order additional copies of *Complications: A Doctor's Love Story*:

Send check to: Linda Gromko MD
Bainbridge Books
200 W. Mercer #104
Seattle, WA 989119

	Price	Quantity	Subtotal
Complications: A Doctor's Love Story	$15.00		
Shipping and Handling *For the first book*	$4.00		
Additional Shipping and Handling *For each additonal book*	$1.00		
Sales Tax *(WA State Residents add 9.5%)*			
Total			

Shipping Information:

Name: ______________________________

Address: ______________________________

____

City: ______________ State: ________ Zip Code: __________

If you wish to place a credit card order, please visit Dr. Gromko's website at www.LindaGromkoMD.com.